C000038416

Allergy

A to Z

All rights reserved. No part of this publication may be reproduced, stored in a retrieval system or transmitted in any form or by any means, electronic, mechanical, photocopying, recording or otherwise without the prior permission of the author.

Copyright © 2005   Jane Thurnell-Read

ISBN: 0 9542439 2 7

Published by:

Life-Work Potential
Sea View House
Long Rock
Penzance
Cornwall
TR20 8JF
England

Tel: + 44 (0)1736 719030
Fax: + 44 (0)1736 719040
www.lifeworkpotential.com

Allergy

A to Z

Jane Thurnell-Read

Visit
Jane Thurnell-Read's
web site for the general public
www.healthandgoodness.com
for information, tips and inspiration
for a happier, healthier life

also

www.lifeworkpotential.com
for information for practitioners

(Both web sites have associated free monthly online
newsletters – don't forget to sign up)

Other books by the author:

Health Kinesiology: The Muscle Testing System That Talks To The Body
ISBN 0 9542439 0 0, Life-Work Potential, 2002

The Guide To Geopathic Stress
ISBN 1 84333 529 8, Vega, 2002

Verbal Questioning Skills For Kinesiologists
ISBN 0 9542439 19, Life-Work Potential, 2004

Energy Mismatch
ISBN: 0 9542439 35, Life-Work Potential, 2004

This book is dedicated
to all those individuals
who have made
the world wide web possible

Without you
this would have been
a much more difficult book
to research and write

Contents

Introduction

I first became involved in allergy testing in the early 1980's because of my eldest son, who was then eighteen months old. He had eczema, diarrhoea and was hyperactive. I started reading and became convinced he was allergic to something, but what? The main method of detection suggested in books was fasting for five days and then introducing one food a day to see what happened. This would have been a tough regime for an adult to follow, but it was impossible and highly dangerous for a small child.

Fortunately I came across Touch For Health (TFH), a type of kinesiology for the lay person. This offered muscle testing as an alternative way of testing for food allergies. The system was very simple: food was placed in the mouth or on the body and then muscle response was tested. Through this I found that Jonathan was allergic to wheat and several artificial food colourings. I excluded these from his diet, and his health and behaviour improved dramatically. At the time I was a University lecturer feeling vaguely dissatisfied with work. I was so impressed with Jon's progress that I decided to learn TFH myself. For a while I saw some clients and carried on doing some lecturing. Gradually, as I started to have lots of success testing people for food allergies, I got busier and busier with the allergy testing. I became more and more confident of my ability to help people with a wide range of problems, and eventually decided to stop teaching in order to concentrate solely on this satisfying new career.

Then my second son, Thomas, was born. He had severe asthma. When Tom was six months old, a hospital specialist told me he would have liked to prescribe Tom an inhaler, but that he was too young to use it. He painted a future life dependent on drugs, but I was determined that this would not happen. I had tested Tom extensively for foods and found several foods that he was allergic to. Excluding these from his diet did not improve his asthma, but if I fed them to him after a break without them, he would wheeze as I fed him. (People often react more obviously to an allergen if they have not encountered it for some time.) So I knew what I had found was correct, but even when I excluded the problem foods, he still coughed and produced thick yellow mucus from his nose. People in the street would often turn in surprise when they heard this small baby coughing like an old man with a fifty-a-day smoking habit. I was extremely frustrated – I was helping many of my clients to get well and stay well, but I could not help my own small son. I would lie awake at night listening to him coughing and wheezing in his sleep, and I became more and more obsessed with finding an answer.

Once again I started reading extensively and observing him closely. I became convinced he was allergic to airborne substances. I started to test these sorts of things and found he was severely allergic to moulds and cigarette smoke, and had lesser reactions to other inhaled substances. It was possible to avoid food and keep him away from people who smoked, but mould was a completely different problem. I had found the problem, but I did not have a solution.

Shortly after this I came across intra-dermal testing and desensitisation, and I took Tom to a clinic that used this process. This used dilutions of substances injected under the skin. Tom's health improved rapidly, as it meant we were turning off allergic reactions to those things that it was difficult to avoid. This was a costly, painful and slow process, but I was happy to have something that would help him.

Some time later I went on a course taught by Don Harrison of Ffynnonwen Natural Therapy Centre, and I learnt about homeopathic desensitising drops. This worked really well, and Tom became very healthy. I also used it with the thousands of people who came to see me for allergy testing: I used muscle testing to establish the allergy, and then homeopathic desensitisation to turn off the reaction.

In 1987 I went on a health kinesiology course and learnt another way of stopping allergic reactions that could be done simply and easily during the session. By now Tom and Jon were so well that they rarely needed help in this way, but I used the procedures taught in health kinesiology with my clients and saw many amazing results.

Over the years I have tested many people with a wide range of health problems, and found that sorting out allergies/intolerances can make a dramatic and sustained difference to many people's health.

This book contains the knowledge I have gained from allergy testing literally thousands of people, and also a lot of detailed research I have done specifically with this project in mind.

In researching this book I became even more aware of the mass experiment that we are conducting with our health. So many chemicals that are not present in nature are put into our food, our personal care products, our cosmetics, our homes, and the air we breathe. It is easy to blame 'them' for this – the big corporations, but we all have a responsibility. As long as we demand food that is available all year round, that is cheap and convenient, as long as we seek 'new' products without looking at the impact of them on our environment this experiment will continue. This book is not about the danger of these chemicals, rather it focuses on the potential for allergy, but I am certain that as long as we (the public) buy products that can only be produced using so many chemicals, allergy problems will continue to increase.

Most of this book is suitable for both the general reader, and for people with a professional interest in allergies. Appendix 4 deals with issues of specific concern for therapists.

Where words and phrases are in *italics* this indicates that there is a specific entry for that item elsewhere in the book.

What Is Allergy?

The word 'allergy' was first coined by an Austrian paediatrician, Baron Clemens von Pirquet, in 1906 from the Greek 'allos' meaning altered or changed and 'ergon' meaning reaction. So the word 'allergy' literally means 'altered reaction'. He noticed that patients who had received injections of horse serum or smallpox vaccine usually had quicker, more severe reactions to second injections. He used the word allergy to describe the reactions – an altered reaction to something in the environment.

There are still some medical practitioners, usually called clinical ecologists, who use this definition, but in the 1920's the definition of allergy was narrowed or, depending on your point of view, made more rigorous, in mainstream medicine. An emphasis was put on immune system involvement, and reactions where the immune system could not be shown to be involved were excluded. The British Medical Association's 'Complete Family Health Encyclopedia' defines 'allergy' as:

> A collection of conditions caused by inappropriate or exaggerated reaction of the immune system to a variety of substances.

So, allergens are substances that produce a reaction in susceptible individuals, whereas the vast majority of people do not respond in this way. Also, (and critically in this narrowed definition), in allergic reactions the over-reaction of the immune system leads to tissue damage and impaired function rather than immunity.

In the 1960's this definition was refined again to specify the part of the immune system that is involved: immunoglobulin E (IgE). In order to establish if someone has an allergic reaction to a substance (according to this definition) antibodies are looked for in the blood. White blood cells produce IgE antibodies which bind to foreign substances in the body – in this case an allergen. The IgE with its attached allergen then binds to specialised white blood cells (mast cells and basophils), and this causes the release of histamine. Histamine narrows bronchi in lungs, increases permeability of blood vessels, lowers blood pressure, causes itching and stimulates production of acid in the stomach – all typical symptoms of certain types of allergic reaction.

At one time, if an immune system involvement could not be shown, the 'allergic' reaction was often ignored or discounted as insignificant by the medical profession, in spite of the distress to the sufferer. Now, however, many medical practitioners distinguish between allergy and sensitivity. In the case of sensitivity the reaction is not believed to be mediated by the immune system, and symptoms often do not appear immediately on exposure, or may be intermittent even with constant exposure.

A more holistic definition of allergy recognises allergy as leading to a disturbance of the body's natural flow and balance of meridian energy even from exposure to a small amount of a substance. In my practice I use the Health Kinesiology definition produced by Jimmy Scott Ph.D. He defines allergy as:

> … any energy disturbance in response to exposure to a substance. The substance could be a food, cosmetic, chemical, animal hair, pollen, mold, etc…With allergy the energy system reacts to *any* amount of the substance.

Another word you will hear is 'intolerance'. This is sometimes used interchangeably with sensitivity, but sometimes it has a different meaning. In my practice I use intolerance to mean that the person has a problem with the quantity of the substance they encounter. In this definition the person only has a reaction when they exceed their tolerance level for that substance.

We probably all have tolerance levels for everything we are in contact with, but if your tolerance level for oranges, say, is twenty oranges a day, you would probably be unaware that you had a limited tolerance. However, if your tolerance for oranges is one small orange a day, every time you have a large orange you would have some sort of symptom. Also if you have orange marmalade for breakfast, and then a small orange during the morning you would still have a problem.

You can see that the terms 'allergy', 'tolerance' and 'sensitivity' are far from clear, and are used by different groups of people to mean different things. It is important that you are clear what meaning(s) you and anyone you are talking to are using.

In her excellent book 'The Allergy Bible' Linda Gamblin gives this advice to patients who want to communicate well with their medical practitioners:

> The important thing is to get along well and communicate clearly with doctors …Just describing how you react – the actual symptoms – is usually the best approach.… 'sensitive' is usually a much more diplomatic choice than 'allergic'.

Whatever the definitions, many people know that they are worse if they come into contact with specific substances. It is easy to dismiss this view as neurotic and 'all in the mind', if you have not experienced at first hand the effect of these reactions.

Why Do People Become Allergic, And Why Are Allergies On The Increase?

It is often unclear why a person has a tendency to be allergic or intolerant to a range of substances. Medical practitioners talk about 'atopic individuals' - atopic means 'out of place'. To the unknowing this sounds like a medical diagnosis, but in fact all it means is: You have a tendency to have allergies; you may have several different symptoms caused by your allergic reactions; this often runs in families; we don't know why. Describing someone as an atopic individual is not saying anything the person does not already know about themself!

Genetic Predisposition
Allergy problems undoubtedly do run in families, so there may be a genetic component, although the exact mechanism is not clearly understood. Some small genetic mutation can cause the immune system to be triggered more easily, so that family members sharing this mutation will all have a tendency to allergic reactions, although not necessarily to the same substances.

Severe Virus Infections
A severe virus infection can lead to damage to the immune system, so that the individual is more likely to develop allergies in the future.

Parasites
One allergy theory now being proposed is that the lack of the proper enemies (liver fluke, tapeworms, etc.) has led to an idle immune system finding inappropriate work in allergic reactions. There are many antibodies produced in the body to protect it against invasion by harmful organisms. IgE antibodies deal effectively and quickly with the extreme danger of infection by large parasites, such as

tapeworms. Parasites' effect on health can be devastating, so over the years individuals with efficient IgE mechanisms have lived to reproduce and pass on their genes at a greater rate than people with a less efficient IgE mechanism. The IgE antibodies are also involved in allergic and hypersensitivity reactions, so people with these inherited efficient IgE mechanisms are more likely to suffer allergy problems than people who have inherited a less efficient system. This super-charged immune system was a plus for an asthma sufferer's distant ancestors inhabiting a world with many life-threatening parasites, but now leads to a 'trigger-happy' immune system firing off inappropriately.

Other practitioners (notably Hulda Clark in 'Cure For All Diseases') take the opposite view, and see many allergy symptoms as being a reaction to an infestation of parasites.

Excessive Cleanliness

The obsession with the danger of 'germs' is thought to have led to an increase in allergies. Much of this obsession with cleanliness seems to be driven by the media and advertising. Headlines about 'killer bugs', and advertisements that claim a product kills even more germs have led many people to buy more and more products to wipe out these dangerous enemies. A view now gaining ground among many researchers and some doctors is that a certain level of dirt is good for us, particularly during infancy and early childhood when the immune system is maturing.

T-helper cells in the immune system recognise foreign antigens and then secrete substances to activate other cells to fight the invader. In pregnancy the T-helper cells that attack invaders directly without producing antibodies (Th1 cells) are less active, as these could lead the mother's system to reject the foetus. This means that the T-helper cells that are responsible for antibody reactions (Th2 cells) are more prominent. These are the ones that are involved in allergic reactions. The new baby's immune system has the same emphasis as the mother's had during pregnancy. It is believed that the exposure of the very young to some level of 'dirt' is beneficial in that it helps to rebalance the immune system to emphasise the T-helper cells that are not involved in the allergy process.

In an excellent article ('New Scientist' July 18th 1998) Garry Hamilton talks about 'the gentler side of germs'. If the young are not exposed to 'dirt', the immune system does not go through this rebalancing process, and a tendency to allergy can result. Linda Gamblin in 'The Allergy Bible' cites several medical research projects, which support the idea of allowing children to be exposed to dirt and minor infections to help protect against allergies.

Vaccination
Our children are now being vaccinated against a bigger and bigger range of diseases. While some of these are serious, many are mild illnesses that were once considered part of a normal childhood. Many alternative practitioners consider that these childhood illnesses help to prime the immune system so that it is better able to cope with a whole range of illnesses later in life. This view is not accepted by most of the medical profession, and indeed it would be difficult to prove. However, there is some evidence that vaccination alters the ratio of T-helper cells and T-suppresser cells. This would be likely to have an effect on the vaccinated child's susceptibility to allergy reactions. It is also known that most vaccines stimulate the branch of the immune system that is concerned with the more extreme immune reactions to invaders such as parasites ('New Scientist' July 18th 1998).

Ubiquitous Presence Of Some Foods
Before the advent of freezers and airfreight most people ate local foods in season. Now most fruit and vegetables are available all year round, so that our systems are exposed to the same foods continually without respite.

There has been a dramatic increase in people experiencing *soya* allergy, since soya has become a common ingredient in many processed foods. In Europe and North America rice allergy is relatively uncommon, whereas in Asia where it is consumed more frequently it is much more common.

Technological Developments

Developments that make modern life more comfortable have also led to an increase in allergies. With the advent of air conditioning, central heating and wall-to-wall carpeting house dust mites and moulds such as alternaria have an ideal environment in which to thrive. Modern offices with sealed windows mean that everyone is exposed to the perfumes worn by other people. The increasing use of plastics, formaldehyde, benzene etc. have led to all of us being exposed to an amazing variety of chemicals.

Contamination By Environmental Pollutants

The chemicals in diesel fumes are known to damage the outer membranes of pollens. This means that when the pollen is breathed in, the pollen proteins are immediately in much closer contact with the delicate membranes in the mouth, nose and lungs than they would be if the pollen had not been damaged in this way.

It has now also been suggested that the immune system is reacting to some harmless substances because they have been contaminated by environmental pollution: the immune system does not recognise the food, for example, if it has molecules from tyre rubber attached to it. These molecules sometimes appear similar to enzymes produced by parasites and so the immune system attacks the 'parasite'.

Although more and more evidence is accumulating for a role for environmental pollutants, this does not explain why New Zealand, which is relatively unpolluted, has one of the highest incidences of asthma in the world.

Electro-Magnetic Pollution

An increase in electro-magnetic pollution has run parallel with the increase in allergies. The scientific jury is still out on the danger of mobile phones, power lines, etc., but many people are becoming more concerned about our constant exposure. See my book 'Geopathic Stress' for more information on this. People who are sensitive to computers, etc. often also show many symptoms typical of allergic individuals. In some cases correcting this sensitivity to electro-magnetic sources, results in all or most of the adverse reactions disappearing. (I recommend health kinesiology for this – see page 50.)

Stress

The pace of life is quickening all the time: modern technology gives us more possibilities and many of us want to experience as many of these as we can. A survey ('Daily Telegraph' December 9th 1999) found that half of the 950 young people in their 20's interviewed said that they would feel a failure if they did not own a home by 26, were not married by 27 and not both rich and parents by 29. Many of the interviewees said they were prepared to sacrifice a healthy diet and way of life to achieve this. These expectations and pressures are not conducive to long-term health and can also lead to stress and allergies. Pre-packaged, processed foods eaten in front of the television, too much alcohol, too little fresh air and exercise all take their toll.

Sometimes particular traumatic events can explain a particular allergy. One of my clients was allergic to wool and tea. She told me that when she was a small child she had pulled a cup of hot tea on to herself. At the time she was wearing a wool sweater, and the tea soaked into the sweater and burnt her very badly.

Diet

It is now well known that bottle-fed babies are more likely to be prone to allergy problems than breast-fed ones. Sudden or early weaning can contribute to the problem too.

Sadly the modern diet may be abundant in calories, but there is more and more evidence that it is low in some important nutrients. People are eating more pre-processed foods, which may be nutritionally compromised.

Soil is becoming depleted of some minerals, because they have long been taken up by plants grown in the soil. If the mineral is not in the soil, it cannot be in the plant, and so it is not available in the foods we eat either.

It is unlikely that there is one simple answer as to why people are allergic, intolerant or sensitive in general or to particular substances. Research is still being carried out in this fascinating area. Fortunately with the tools that are available it is not necessary to know why someone has allergy problems in order to be able to detect and correct them.

Allergy Equals Addiction

Craving particular foods can be a sign of a need for a nutrient that is in the food that is craved. The body is demanding food that contains a particular nutrient. This can be very straight-forward. For example, I spent three months in Sri Lanka, and my diet was very short of zinc. The moment I walked back into my house I reached for the jar of sunflower seeds (an excellent source of zinc) and started stuffing them down myself. Over the next few days I ate a huge amount of sunflower seeds. Initially I really craved them, but after a few days the obsession disappeared. It was only with hindsight that I realised why I had done that.

When petrol contained lead, I had several clients who ate a lot of apples, but testing using kinesiology showed they were not allergic to them. It took me a while to realise why. Most of them were allergic to petrol, which probably meant they were less able to deal with the lead in it than someone who was not allergic to petrol. Apples contain pectin, which is an excellent chelator of lead, (i.e. it can remove lead from the body), so it seemed that these people were instinctively reaching for the pectin to counteract the lead in the petrol.

However, cravings are more likely to indicate an allergy problem. Allergy often seems to equal addiction and the reason for this is not totally clear. It has been suggested that this may be because some protein fragments formed when food is broken down are similar to endorphins, which the body produces naturally to counteract pain and produce euphoria. Then the allergy sufferer's body becomes adapted to that level of endorphin activity and so craves the allergen in order to maintain the endorphin levels.

One indication of a possible allergy problem is waking with a 'hangover' when alcohol has not been consumed the night before. This very often points to one or more food allergies. The person eats the food during the day and satisfies the craving, but during the night withdrawal symptoms begin, and classically the person wakes with a 'hangover'. Eating the allergen switches off the withdrawal symptoms and allows the person to feel better. In fact some people will not make it through the night without having a snack of their allergen in the early hours to keep their withdrawal symptoms at bay. They are often totally surprised when told that they are reacting to the very food they like and experience as making them feel better.

Because of the addictive nature of allergies some people may have difficulty losing weight. There are two possible scenarios. Firstly they could be allergic to some high calorie food and find it extremely difficult to moderate their consumption because they are addicted to it. The second possibility is that the person experiences withdrawal symptoms, but for some reason does not seem to connect the withdrawal symptoms with a particular food. In this case they keep on eating different foods without feeling satisfied. They only stop when they consume the allergen, but the turning off of the craving only usually lasts for a short time. Overall calorie consumption can be very high in these people even if the allergen is lettuce. In any event allergy-induced addictions can lead to bingeing and an inability to control food intake.

Because of this allergy-driven addiction problem, some people will like smells that most people do not, e.g. creosote and petrol/gas. Almost invariably the person is allergic to this, and is getting their 'fix'. Teenagers who sniff glue may be allergic to it, and while counselling may be necessary, correcting this allergy will almost certainly help enormously.

A child with a lot of food sensitivities will often be a fussy eater. The parent will frequently say: 'My child would be happy if he/she could live on X.' The child is probably allergic to X, whatever that is. Frequently they become irritable and bad-tempered if they have to go without their favourite food for even a short period of time. Breast fed babies with allergies are usually either difficult feeders or need to be constantly fed both day and night and may be difficult to wean.

Some years ago I had a funny example of the allergic addiction phenomenon. I went to visit a friend, who had a cat. When I went into the kitchen I saw cat food scattered over quite an area around the cat's food bowl. My friend explained that her cat was a very untidy eater, and she had not had time to clear it up before my visit. I knew that in general cats were tidy eaters, so I wondered if the cat was desperately searching through its dinner for the particular food it craved. I did some testing and found several allergies. I corrected the problems, and after that the cat became a tidy eater like all the other cats I know.

What Symptoms Can Be
The Result Of Allergies?

It is easy to be over-influenced by the current medical understanding and only think about allergy in relation to a limited numbers of illnesses, such as asthma, eczema and hay fever.

I had a very salutary experience in the early days of my practice. At that time I was working exclusively with allergy problems, and a lady phoned me and asked to make an appointment, as she was suffering from trigeminal neuralgia. I told her that I did not know of any evidence for an allergy link for this painful complaint and persuaded her not to come to see me. A week later she phoned again and was most insistent on seeing me. Once again I explained my reservations, but agreed to see her. Testing showed she was allergic to *lead*, which she was exposed to in her work – she made small pewter boxes. We dealt with the problem, and she made a very rapid recovery.

Another client came to me after having been diagnosed as suffering from post-natal depression. Testing showed she was highly allergic to *formaldehyde*. I told her the most common sources of formaldehyde, which include cavity wall insulation. She replied that her house had been insulated two weeks before her symptoms had started. Although I was able to desensitise her to this, she decided to move house. She later told me: 'That house has caused me so much misery. My family were very close to admitting me to a mental hospital because I was so ill, and within one week of moving I feel happy and contented again.'

A small child, who was brought to see me because she wet her bed in the summer only, turned out to be allergic to *pollens*. Once we had corrected this the bed-wetting stopped completely.

Many different symptoms and illnesses can be caused by an allergic reaction or have an allergy component. What follows is not a complete list, but is intended to give some understanding of the breadth of problems that can have an allergy/intolerance component.

For some of the entries I have included likely culprits, but it is essential to be completely open-minded, because the basic rule is anything can cause a problem for anybody.

IT IS IMPORTANT TO REMEMBER THAT MANY OF THESE SYMPTOMS CAN HAVE CAUSES OTHER THAN THAT OF ALLERGY OR INTOLERANCE.

Abdominal Pain And/Or Bloating
Persistent abdominal pain and/or bloating can be as a result of many different factors, but one very common possibility is allergy/intolerance reactions. A common culprit is *wheat*.

Acne
Allergies exacerbate a pre-existing condition in some people.

ADD
See *attention deficit disorder*.

Addictions
See page 13.

Adhesions
Sometimes the fibrin strands that form after surgery do not dissolve, but become permanent, forming thick bands linking organs that were previously separate. This leads to pain, because organs are restricted in their movement, and nerve fibres are stretched. Adhesions most commonly occur after pelvic/gynaecological

surgery. Some research has suggested that this can occur as a result of *latex* sensitivity, as the surgeons wear gloves made of latex.

Alcoholism

There is undoubtedly a genetic pre-disposition to alcoholism, and in some families and cultures *alcohol* is seen as being a perfectly reasonable way of dealing with all sorts of stresses and crises, but an allergy to one or more of the components of alcoholic drinks can exacerbate any tendency. The allergy to the ingredient(s) - commonly *brewer's yeast*, *grapes*, *hops*, *malt*, *grains* or any of the processing chemicals – leads to addictive drinking, which fuels an underlying tendency to alcoholism.

Allergic Rhinitis

This involves inflammation of the mucous membranes that line the nasal passages. Symptoms may include itching of the nose, roof of the mouth, eyes and throat. Some people also suffer from sneezing, runny nose and watering eyes. Common problem substances include *house dust, house dust mite, pollens, animal hair, moulds, perfumes, bleach, solvents, tobacco smoke* and *vehicle exhaust fumes*.

Anaphylactic Shock

A life-threatening allergic reaction. Massive amounts of *histamine* and other chemicals are released, causing immediate changes to body tissues: the blood vessels dilate causing a sudden lowering of blood pressure, and swelling of the tongue and airways occurs. *Peanuts*, shellfish and *bee stings* are common culprits. Tryptase is an enzyme released during anaphylaxis, which can be measured on a blood test to confirm that this type of allergic reaction has definitely occurred. See also *angioedema*.

Angioedema

This is similar to *urticaria*, but affects the body at the level of the blood vessels, causing swelling from excess fluid. Often caused by a sudden reaction to seafood, *peanuts*, strawberries or *eggs*. Common sites are the skin, the gastro-intestinal tract and the throat and larynx. This can be very dangerous causing difficulty in breathing, speaking and swallowing. During an attack emergency medical treatment is likely to be needed. Often involved in *anaphylactic shock*. Common culprits are *bee sting*, *penicillin*, *aspirin*, *food colourings* and preservatives, shellfish, strawberries, *nuts* and *peanuts*.

Anxiety
Anxiety with its feeling of fear often has a psychological base, but allergies can be a precipitating or exacerbating factor too, particularly to *coffee*, *tea*, *chocolate*, *food colourings* and other chemicals.

Arrhythmia
This is when the heart has an irregular or abnormal heart beat. Many different substances can cause this problem. Excess *coffee* consumption can cause the same problem, and this may be either an allergic reaction or a straight-forward physiological reaction to the amount of *caffeine*, a central nervous system stimulant, that is consumed.

Aspergillosis
This is a reaction to the fungus *Aspergillus fumigatus*, which is found in soil and dust and decaying vegetable matter. In some people the spores grow in the lung mucus, causing an allergic reaction.

Asthma
Sometimes asthma starts after a virus infection - often respiratory synctial virus (RSV). Many different substances can trigger an asthma attack. Common culprits include *dairy products*, *food colourings*, *formaldehyde*, *house dust mite*, *pollens*, *pet hair* and *moulds*. Some asthma has also been linked to chronic trichophyton diseases such as athlete's foot. The body is producing IgE antibodies

in an attempt to fight the athlete's foot; the antibodies are carried in the blood stream to the respiratory system, and symptoms of asthma may appear. See also *urticaria*.

Attention Deficit Disorder (ADD)

Children who are unable to concentrate, and are clumsy and very restless. There is some evidence that ADD children tend to turn into depressed adults unless the condition is rectified. In my experience of treating children with this complaint, if allergies play a large part in the problem, then the child almost always has other physical symptoms too (often *eczema* or *asthma*). Common culprits include *food colourings* and other chemicals.

Autism

This sometimes responds to allergy/intolerance work.

Bad Breath

Bad breath may be a symptom of poor oral hygiene, gum disease or digestive problems. Digestive problems often have an allergic component so allergies are worth considering for this embarrassing problem.

Bed Wetting

See *incontinence*.

Bingeing

Allergy induced cravings can lead to bingeing and inappropriate eating patterns. See page 13.

Blood Sugar Levels

See *hypoglycaemia*.

Brain Fog

Many people with allergies feel as though their brains are not working properly. Foods may be the culprits but so may inhaled chemicals, particularly *formaldehyde*.

Bronchitis

While smoking is the main cause of chronic bronchitis, allergies may be the problem or a contributing factor for some people. *Cigarette smoke* (including passive inhalation), *house dust mite*, *moulds* and *pollens* are the most likely problems, but not the only ones.

Burping

This is usually accompanied by other symptoms when it is allergy based.

Candidiasis

The condition caused by Candida albicans. Candida albicans is normally a harmless yeast organism present in the human gut, where it lives in balance with the normal bacterial population of the gut. Sometimes the number of Candida albicans organisms increases dramatically, and the way in which the organism grows changes. It has been suggested that when Candida proliferates it is able to change the way in which it grows, and it can permeate the walls of the intestine and allow food molecules to pass into the body producing allergic responses to these foods. Many people who have this problem are also allergic to the Candida organism itself.

This over-growth of Candida can be caused by, for example, antibiotics (directly affecting the bacteria balance in the gut), steroids (suppressing the body's immune system), hormonal changes in pregnancy, use of the contraceptive pill, and poor diets high in refined carbohydrate and sugar.

Symptoms include *bloating*, *diarrhoea*, itchy anus and *fatigue*. Many doctors are sceptical about the role of Candida albicans in this combination of symptoms. Many complementary therapists seem to believe that these symptoms are always attributable to Candida problems. In fact, these symptoms can also be triggered by other allergies, and by other problems entirely, but it is always worth checking out Candida. Other Candida strains (such as Candida glabrata and Candida krusei) are becoming an increasing problem.

Car/Automobile Sickness
This often indicates problems with *vehicle exhaust fumes*. It can also indicate a reaction to *moulds* in cars with *air conditioning systems*. In newer cars it may also indicate a problem with *plastics*, etc.

Catarrh
This is inflammation of mucous membranes with a production of excessive amounts of mucus. It may lead to *sinusitis*, *rhinitis* or *otitis media*.

Celiac Disease
See *coeliac disease*.

Chinese Restaurant Syndrome
Symptoms include flushing, sweating, and headaches. The common culprit *is monosodium glutamate*, but there are other possibilities such as fish sauce.

Coeliac Disease
Also known as gluten-sensitivity entropathy or non-tropical sprue. An inflammatory disease of the intestine, with damage to the villi of the intestine leading to malabsorption, caused by a reaction to *gluten*. Typical symptoms include extreme tiredness, weight loss and *diarrhoea*. Damage to the intestinal wall can allow other food molecules through, setting off further reactions to other foods. There are genetic factors involved particularly where coeliac disease

starts early in a child's life. Coeliac disease can start as an adult, when an underlying genetic tendency is exacerbated by some environmental trigger. The genetic predisposition involves the body producing antibodies to one of its own enzymes, that is involved in the breakdown of gluten in the intestine. Where coeliac disease runs in families, some members may suffer from *dermatitis herpetiformis* instead. It is important to realise that not everyone who reacts to *wheat* is a coeliac or sensitive to gluten.

Colic, Infantile
A severe abdominal pain leading the infant to scream and pull up its legs. Allergy/intolerance problems (particularly to *lactose*) are always worth checking in this situation, although there can be other causes too. If the baby is unwell between bouts of colic, this could indicate a more serious illness. Babies with parents who smoke are much more prone to colic, but it is unclear why this is the case.

Colitis
Inflammation of the colon often responds well to allergy work. One of the most common culprits is *wheat*, but be aware that wheat may exacerbate the symptoms not because of an allergy, but because the bran in the wheat irritates the membranes of the colon which are already inflamed for other reasons.

Conjunctivitis
Also known as pink eye. It is inflammation of the membrane that lines the inside of the eyelid and touches the white part of the eye, resulting in soreness and irritation. It can be part of a *hay fever* syndrome, along with sneezing and a runny nose. One of my clients developed severe conjunctivitis every time she was anywhere near anyone wearing *acrylic* fake fur. This can also be caused by an infection.

Constipation

Occasionally caused by an allergy, often to *cow's milk*, particularly if associated with *wheezing* and/or *eczema*.

Contact Dermatitis

See *dermatitis*.

Coughing

Coughing is an attempt to clear the airways, and can be indicative of a variety of problems, including allergies. See also *post-nasal drip*.

Cravings

See Allergy Equals Addiction page 13.

Crohn's Disease

A chronic inflammatory disease affecting part of the digestive tract – usually the small or large intestine. Symptoms can include pain, fever, weight loss and *diarrhoea*. Common culprits are *wheat* and *dairy* products.

Dark Circles Or Bags Under The Eyes

These make the person look permanently tired. In Chinese medicine this area of the face is linked to the adrenal glands. The adrenal glands are one of the main organs of the body involved in stress reactions and exposure to allergens certainly produces stress in the body. The crease seen under the eyelids of some allergy sufferers is referred to as a Dennie Line.

Depression

Although depression often has an emotional or biochemical basis, allergies may be a contributing or precipitating factor.

Dermatitis

The skin becomes inflamed and will be sore and possibly itchy. Contact dermatitis occurs when the skin reacts to something it is in contact with, such as *nickel, chromium, perfume,* some plants and *latex.* Sometimes the dermatitis appears in a sensitive area of the skin rather than the actual site of the initial contact. For example, a *nail polish* allergy may not show up on the robust skin around the nail, but could affect the more sensitive skin around the eyes, because it has been touched by the varnished nail. Can also be caused by reactions to commonly consumed foods.

Dermatitis Herpetiformis
In families where *coeliac disease* is common some members may experience this reaction to *gluten.* Symptoms include a chronic, symmetrical, itchy rash. Common areas are the back, buttocks, elbows, knees and scalp.

Dermatographism
Some allergy sufferers have a skin that is highly sensitive and reactive and will develop a red line or an itchy weal if the skin is firmly stroked. It is a form of *urticaria.*

Diarrhoea
Diarrhoea can occur for many reasons, some of them life-threatening, so this should never be treated lightly. Reactions to food can lead to diarrhoea. The length of time that elapses between the consumption of the food and the start of the diarrhoea varies from person to person. In some people the reaction occurs long before the offending food could physically have reached the intestine.

Diverticulitis
This is inflammation of the diverticula of the colon. Many different foods can be involved. Some people believe that they are allergic to wholemeal *wheat* flour because of the pain etc. they experience when they eat products made from wholemeal flour. This may not be an allergic reaction, but a physical reaction caused by the irritation of the inflamed area by the rough bran in wholemeal flour.

Drowsiness

Drowsiness can be a sign of a life-threatening situation, but habitual drowsiness after meals can be a sign that the person is consuming something in the meals to which they are allergic.

Dry Or Flaky Lips

Judging by the amount of *lip balm* that is sold many people suffer from dry or flaky lips. Sometimes the edge of the lip is an indistinct blur rather than there being a definite line between it and the rest of the face. Michio Kushi in his book 'Oriental Diagnosis' says that different parts of the lip correspond to different parts of the digestive system: the upper lip represents the stomach; the lower part corresponds to the intestines. These parts of the body are often involved with allergic reactions particularly if the problem is with foods. See also *lip balm*.

Earache and Ear Infections

See *otitis media*.

Eczema

Common culprits are *cow's milk, house dust mite, detergents, perfumes*, man-made fibres (such as *polyester* and *acrylic*), *lanolin, nickel* and *pet hair*. Can be triggered by airborne allergens in some people. This may be because some of the airborne particles are swallowed rather than inhaled.

Sometimes people will show eczema in different places depending on what they have been exposed to. For example, my eldest son used to get eczema in the flexures of his legs and arms whenever he ate *wheat*, but if he ate something with the food colouring *tartrazine* in it he would get a small patch of eczema in one specific place on his back, whereas another food colouring would make him itch at a different spot on his back. As far as I know this is an individual thing, so wheat or these food colourings could cause someone else to itch in a different place. This may explain why sometimes eczema is successfully cleared from some places on the body, but not from others – the allergen(s) that apply to only some areas have been successfully dealt with.

Sometimes eczema appears in a particular area because of direct contact with an allergen. A client whose eczema was so severe he had been hospitalised on several occasions told me that the only time the eczema on his legs cleared was when he went into hospital. I found he was allergic to the *indigo* dye in the jeans he always wore, which suggested that it was not the hospital treatment itself, but simply that in hospital he wore pyjamas all day rather than jeans.

As an added complication, fungal and bacterial infections can colonise the skin legions in eczema, causing further irritation. When this is the case, removing the allergens that started the eczema will not be sufficient to allow the skin to settle down. The micro-organisms involved are usually Staphylococcus aureus, Candida or Trichophyton.
If fungal infection of the eczema is a problem, there will usually be scarring or the skin will look silvery as it heals.

Eczema sufferers will sometimes also react to Pityrosporum ovale. This is a yeast that is normally present on the surface of the skin.

Enuresis
See *incontinence*.

Fatigue
Abnormal tiredness, often accompanied by *hypoglycaemia* and *mood swings*, may be a sign of allergy problems.

Flatulence
Flatulence leads to abdominal discomfort, and there may also be embarrassment when the wind is passed. Usually a sign of digestive disturbance, which may indicate allergy problems.

Fluid Retention
See *oedema*.

Flushing
Facial flushing may be a reaction to consuming or coming into contact with an allergen. The reaction is usually immediate.

Food Cravings
See Allergy Equals Addiction page 13.

Fungal Infections
Mostly commonly *candidiasis* (thrush) and tinea (ringworm and athletes foot). Often people are allergic to the fungus, and so the body is less able to deal with it.

Glue Ear
See *otitis media*.

Halitosis
See *bad breath*.

Hard Skin On The Feet
Most people get some hard skin on their feet, but some people get an excessive amount. This sometimes becomes less after allergies have been corrected. Reflexology has shown that zones on the feet are linked to specific parts of the body, so it may be that the calluses grow in order to shield organ reflex areas, and disappears when this is no longer necessary.

Hay Fever
The common name for one type of *allergic rhinitis*. An allergy caused by *pollen*. Affects the delicate lining of the nose, eyes and roof of the mouth. Many people mistake the symptoms of hay fever for a 'summer cold'. In Western Europe the mould *Cladosporium herbarum* produces spores in June, so some people who show

classic hay fever symptoms at the classic time may be reacting to this mould either as well as pollen or rather than pollen.

The peak season for hay fever in the UK is May/June, but some sufferers will start in February or March and go through to September/October. See Appendix C for a pollen calendar. Incidences of hay fever have increased dramatically in cities, and it has been found that *pollution* can strip the outer membrane off the pollen spore making contact with the pollen itself more potent.

Headache
Allergens are a common cause of headaches. See also *migraine*.

Hives
See *urticaria*.

Hyperactivity
See *attention deficit disorder*.

Hyperkinetic Syndrome
See *attention deficit disorder*.

Hypoglycaemia
Some people have unstable blood sugar levels, caused by a reaction to food(s) they eat. The allergen causes a rapid increase in blood sugar followed by a dramatic fall, a classic hypoglycaemic effect. The foods involved are not necessarily ones that normally trigger a rapid rise in blood sugar.

IBS
See *irritable bowel syndrome*.

Incontinence, Urinary
Uncontrollable, involuntary passing of urine can occasionally be attributable to an allergic reaction.

Indigestion

Indigestion is a bit of a catch-all term, covering various symptoms, such as heartburn, *abdominal bloating, flatulence* and *nausea*, indicating a problem within the digestive system. May be solely or partially attributable to allergies.

Irritable Bowel Syndrome

A combination of intermittent *abdominal pain* and irregular bowel habits, involving *constipation, diarrhoea* (or both) in the absence of other diagnosed disease. Also known as spastic colon. A recent study suggested that *yeast* was the main culprit, with *wheat*, peas, cashew nuts, almonds, *barley*, beef and *soya* also being frequent problems.

Irritability

Often seen as a psychological problem, but some allergy sufferers will suffer in this way either as a direct allergic reaction, or as a result of experiencing withdrawal symptoms (see page 13).

Itching

Common culprits include *tartrazine, drugs, nickel* and occupational chemicals.

Migraine

Migraine symptoms include vision disturbances and/or *nausea* and *vomiting* as well as a severe *headache*. Many migraine sufferers react to high levels of tyramine in food. This is not necessarily an allergic reaction. Tyramine raises the blood pressure, and migraine sufferers have been shown to be slower as excreting tyramine than non-migraine sufferers. Common triggers are *chocolate, cheese,* citrus fruit, *coffee, alcohol* (particularly red wine), meat extract, stock cubes and nitrates in processed meat.

Mood swings
These can in some cases be a reaction to allergies. This is usually because of the allergens effect on the blood sugar, and so on the brain.

Morning 'Hangovers'
People who frequently wake feeling as though they have a hangover when they have not been drinking alcohol are likely to be suffering from either low blood sugar or else allergy problems. See also Allergy Equals Addiction page 13.

ME
See *post-viral syndrome.*

Mouth ulcers
These are open sores caused by a break in the mucous membranes of the mouth. Foods, *toothpaste*, *lipstick* and *alcohol* are common culprits.

Multiple Chemical Sensitivities
Where an individual is sensitive to a number of environmental chemicals. Symptoms commonly include *headaches*, *fatigue*, skin conditions, *runny nose*, *vomiting* and *diarrhoea*. Individuals, such as painters, printers, hairdressers and carpet fitters are particularly susceptible, because they are exposed repeatedly to a small range of chemicals in their work. This often leads to a more generalised sensitivity to a whole range of common chemicals.

Myalgic Encephalomyelitis
See *post-viral syndrome.*

Nasal Congestion
See *catarrh.*

Nausea
Usually if an allergy is the problem it is easy to identify, because the response is so immediate. See also *vomiting*.

Nettle Rash
See *urticaria*.

Obesity
See page 14.

Oedema
An abnormal accumulation of fluid in body tissues can be a direct result of exposure to one or more allergens. If the fluid retention varies with the menstrual cycle, it is less likely to be allergy based.

Otitis Media
Low-grade eardrum inflammation associated with fluid in the middle ear cavity. Also known as glue ear. Ears may feel blocked and/or itchy, and the sufferer may experience deafness. If a child has grown up with the problem, he/she may not complain because it is 'normal'. The fluid build up in the ear can be an ideal breeding ground for bacteria, and so result in infection.

Panic Attacks
These often have a psychological basis, but on occasions may be triggered by allergic reactions, either as a direct symptom of the allergy, or as a result of withdrawal symptoms being experienced.

Perennial Allergic Rhinitis
See *allergic rhinitis*.

Persistent Cough
See *coughing*.

Pink Eye
See *conjunctivitis*.

Post-Nasal Drip
Excess mucus produced in the nose runs into the throat and, sometimes, into the airways. This may lead to coughing.

Post-Viral Syndrome
Experienced when someone does not fully recover from a viral infection. Symptoms may include exhaustion, muscle weakness, dizziness, numbness, depression and lack of concentration and motivation. In my clinical practice I have found that these people often have multiple allergy problems, but once the underlying imbalance is corrected (usually viral detoxification and correcting electro-magnetic problems), many of these will disappear.

Rash
See *skin rashes*.

Red Ears
One or both ears red (and sometimes burning) is usually a symptom of allergy, unless the air temperature is particularly cold, in which case red ears are perfectly normal. The reaction usually starts about 1¾ hours after exposure to the offending substance and lasts for about half an hour. This particular reaction can be a very useful self-help diagnostic technique.

Red Eyes
See *conjunctivitis*.

Rhinitis
See *allergic rhinitis*.

Runny Nose
See *catarrh*.

Schizophrenia

Some schizophrenics have responded well to eliminating *gluten* and *milk* from their diet.

Sinusitis

Inflammation of the mucous membranes lining the sinuses in the head. Some recent research has suggested that some sufferers go on to develop allergic reactions to *moulds* that grow in the mucus trapped in the sinuses.

Skin Rashes

Skin rashes can be caused by a wide variety of allergens, including chemicals, *nickel* and *drugs*, particularly *antibiotics*.

Sleep Disturbance

Allergic reactions can be one possible cause of sleep disturbances. The allergen can stimulate the body so that it is difficult to relax and sleep. Also withdrawal symptoms may lead to waking during the night (see page 14).

Sleepiness

See *drowsiness*.

Sneezing

Sneezing usually occurs as a result of irritation of the upper respiratory tract. One cause of this irritation is exposure to an allergen. Having sneezing fits first thing most mornings is often attributable to *house dust mite*.

Sore Throat

Sore throats are often the result of infection, but a persistent sore throat without any other symptoms could indicate allergy problems.

Spastic Colon

See *irritable bowel syndrome*.

Stomach Ache
See *indigestion.*

Summer 'Cold'
Many people will say they have a cold, when in fact they have an allergy to something in the air at that time. A normal cold lasts about a week, but these so-called summer colds will go on for several weeks as long as the particular *pollen* allergen is prevalent in the air.

Sweaty Feet
When the body is burdened with allergic reactions, it may lead to sweaty feet, as a form of detoxification. Correcting the underlying allergies will usually lead to a dramatic improvement in this problem.

Swelling
See *oedema* and *urticaria.*

Tachycardia
A rapid heartbeat can be the result of exposure to an allergen. As this is often immediate, it is usually easy to identify the offending substance.

Tilt
An abbreviation for *toxicant-induced loss of tolerance.*

Tiredness
See *fatigue.*

Total Allergy Syndrome
See *multiple chemical sensitivities.*

Toxicant-Induced Loss Of Tolerance

Also known as Tilt. Another name used in the USA for *multiple chemical sensitivities*.

Urticaria

Also called hives or nettle rash. A condition characterised by an itchy rash consisting of white or yellow lumps surrounded by an area of red inflammation. Common culprits are *food additives*, chemicals, *nickel*, and *drugs*. Some unfortunate people develop urticaria in reaction to sunlight. Chronic urticaria has been linked to chronic trichophyton diseases such as athlete's foot, and chronic sinusitis or throat infections. The body is producing IgE antibodies in an attempt to fight the athlete's foot; the antibodies are carried in the blood stream and symptoms of urticaria may appear elsewhere. See also *asthma*.

Vomiting

This can occur as a result of *angioedema* affecting the digestive tract. See also *nausea*.

Water Retention

See *oedema*.

Wheezing

See *asthma*.

Wind

See *flatulence*.

Allergy Signs In Children

This information is available elsewhere in this book, but it is appropriate to gather it together in one place. Many parents and carers wonder if a child's problems and symptoms could be the result of allergy. The more of the following signs that apply to the child, the more likely it is that his/her problems are at least in part allergy-based.

Dark Circles Or Bags Under The Eyes
These make the child look permanently tired. In Chinese medicine this area of the face is linked to the adrenal glands. The adrenal glands are one of the main organs of the body involved in stress reactions, and exposure to allergens certainly produces stress in the body. Sometimes there is also a crease seen under the eyelids.

Dry, Flaky Lips
Often the edge of the lip is an indistinct blur rather than there being a definite line between it and the rest of the face. Michio Kushi in his book 'Oriental Diagnosis' says that different parts of the lip correspond to different parts of the digestive system. The upper lip represents the stomach. The lower part corresponds to the intestines. These parts of the body are often involved with allergic reactions particularly if the problem is with foods.

Sweaty Feet
The liver is the main detoxifying organ of the body. When it is not functioning properly or has to work overtime then the feet tend to be very sweaty. In allergic reactions the liver is coping with an overload of toxins.

One Or Both Ears Sometimes Red And/Or Burning

This reaction usually starts about 1¾ hours after exposure to the offending substance and lasts for about ½ an hour. I do not know whether it is significant if it is one ear or both ears, but the timing seems very precise. This particular reaction can become a very useful self-help diagnostic technique.

Blond Haired & Pale

Children with a tendency to allergies often have blond hair. They are usually pale; in fact so pale that sometimes they are suspected of suffering from anaemia. In some children this paleness is not at first sight evident, because they have very rosy cheeks either all the time or some of the time. Sometimes the child's cheek will be hot and burning, or papery and dry.

A Fussy Eater

A child with a lot of food sensitivities will often be a fussy eater. The parent will often say: 'My child would be happy if he could live on X.' The child is probably allergic to X, whatever that is. Frequently they become irritable and bad-tempered if they have to go without their favourite food for even a short period of time Breast fed babies are either difficult feeders or need to be constantly fed both day and night and may be difficult to wean.

First Thing In The Morning

Babies and children with food allergies are usually either very good tempered or very bad tempered first thing in the morning.

Family History Of Allergies

Very often there is a family history of allergies with close relatives suffering from eczema, hay fever, etc.

Likes Particular Smells

Allergic children (and adults) often like peculiar smells: they sniff felt tip pens or enjoy the smell of petrol (gas) at petrol stations. They are nearly always allergic to the smell they like so much and, like a drug addict, are seeking out a fix. See also allergy equals addiction page 13.

Correlations

Symptoms Worse At A Particular Time Of the Year

People who develop symptoms at a particular time of the year may be responding to a seasonal allergen. *Pollens* or *moulds* and *heating fumes* fall into this category. I have had clients who have felt they were not allergic to pollens, because their symptoms were not worse in the summer. On testing they were shown to react to moulds and pollens, so their symptoms persisted throughout the year, but they were reacting to different things according to the season. Someone with a tomato allergy will often be driven to see a doctor/therapist in September in the UK (the month may be different elsewhere). At that time of the year tomatoes are very cheap, or there is a glut in the garden, so intake tends to be much higher, and consequently symptoms become so bad that someone with an unsuspected tomato allergy finally decides they need to do something about it.

Symptoms Worse During Or Just After Heavy Rain

There is a dramatic increase in *mould* spores during heavy rain.

Symptoms Worse During Or Just After Thunderstorms

Thunderstorms tend to concentrate *pollen* particles in a narrow band of air close to ground level. There is also a significant increase in *mould* spores in the air.

Symptoms Worse First Thing In The Morning

If symptoms are worse on waking, this will often indicate problems with *detergents*, *house dust mite* or *bedding* fabrics.

Symptoms Worse After Lunch

Many people assume it is normal to feel sleepy after lunch, but this is not the case, unless the lunch was particularly large. Sleepiness at this time of the day will usually indicate a problem with what was eaten at lunchtime.

Symptoms Worse As Day Wears On

This usually suggests that exposure is increasing as the day wears on, so often foods, or else something in the work environment are likely problems.

Symptoms Worse For Exercise

This may be because the exercise involves exposure to some allergen (e.g. in *swimming pool water*, *elastane* in clothing, etc.), or it may be that there is an increased intake of an allergen because of rapid and/or heavy breathing. Sweat on clothes can also mean that detergents etc. that are in exercise clothing may have an enhanced effect. In some people the exertion of exercise can trigger an existing condition (e.g. exercise-induced asthma). This is not necessarily an allergy reaction.

Symptoms Worse At Work

Many different substances at work can cause problems. Common occupational allergens include flour for bakers, and cyanoacrylate *adhesives* for those involved in plastic assembly work. *Latex* gloves are a common problem for doctors, nurses, dentists and their assistants. *Colophony* and *solder* fumes generate allergies for some workers in electronic assembly. Chefs and other kitchen staff may react to cleaning agents and raw fish. Some fishermen react to fish and seaweed. Shampoos and *hair dyes* can affect hairdressers. Wood dust is a problem for some carpenters and saw mill workers.

Symptoms Worse At Home

Pets, home *heating fumes*, *carpets*, etc. may be the problem.

Symptoms Better On Holiday

If symptoms are better at this time it may be because the stress levels are less, so the body is better able to cope with any allergens around, or it could be because exposure to one or more allergens has temporarily ceased.

Symptoms Worse On Holiday Or During Festivities

When people are on holiday or celebrating religious and family holidays, many things change, including food and drink. Festive decorations that are stored from one year to the next can increase exposure to *dust* and *moulds*. Presents may be highly *perfumed* and scented candles can be a problem too. If the vacation or celebrations happen in a completely different environment, the person may be exposed to different airborne substances (*pollens*, *moulds*, industrial *pollution*, etc.). Cleaning chemicals and free personal care products in hotels, etc. may also be a problem.

Detecting Allergies

There are various methods of detecting allergies, and each one has its supporters.

Medical testing seeks to use reproducible tests, i.e. where a repeat test would show exactly the same results even when the tester does not know the original results. *Patch testing*, *skin prick testing* and *scratch testing* are highly reproducible, but are not necessarily accurate, as they only measure the reaction of the skin to a potential allergen. The skin tissues do not necessarily react in the same way as, for example, the lining of the lungs or the stomach. In consequence there are likely to be some false-positive results (i.e. suggesting the person is allergic to something when they are not) or false-negative results (i.e. suggesting the person is not allergic to something when they are).

Other forms of testing, such as *EAV*, *kinesiology* and *radionics testing* may not always pass the medical test of reproducibility, but do have many supporters who recount personal experiences of their accuracy.

I have used health kinesiology (see below) professionally for many years and found it to be a rapid, safe and accurate method of detecting allergies.

Some systems use dilutions of substances for testing. At its simplest this means that a substance is mixed with a solvent, and the resulting liquid is tested. See *intradermal skin testing*, *skin prick testing* and *scratch testing*.

Homeopathic dilutions are used in some systems. This involves diluting the test substance repeatedly, with a sample of the previous dilution being diluted to form the next dilution. This is usually repeated until there is unlikely to be any of the original substance physically present in the liquid, but an 'energy pattern' or memory of the substance is still present. Sometimes a radionics machine is used which magnetically produces the energy pattern of a given substance. Because these do not deteriorate, it allows practitioners to use extensive testing kits. See *electroacupuncture according to Voll*, *kinesiology* and *radionic testing*.

Some systems measure immunoglobulins. These are also known as antibodies. They are produced by the body as part of the immune system. They bind to foreign substances in the body. Each antibody is designed to recognize only a specific antigen. When an antigen is encountered, more copies of the antibody are made. These bind to the antigen, identifying it so that other parts of the immune system attack and destroy it.

There are five main types of antibody: IgA, IgD, IgE, IgG and IgM. Some testing methods are looking at IgE antibodies, whose main function appears to be protecting the body from parasites. See *RAST testing*. Others are checking for IgG antibodies, whose main roles are to protect against bacteria and viruses, and give initial protection to the newborn baby. See *cytotoxic* and *ELISA testing*.

Avoidance & Challenge
Many people will try excluding foods, or changing things in the environment to test out their sensitivity. This can work well, if only a few substances are involved.

The strictest form of this approach involves eating no food and drinking only spring water for 5 days, and then gradually introducing one food at a time. This demands a lot of self-control and does not take into account contact/inhalant allergens or properly allow for tolerance problems. Re-introducing a food after 5 or more days can be very risky as the body may then be in a very sensitive state to that substance. Some authorities recommend that the period of avoidance should be longer before the food is reintroduced.

Of course, it is also possible to remove just one substance at a time. This often works very well, but if it is replaced by something equally problematic then the allergen is not usually identified.

I found that one of my clients had an allergy to pillow feathers, and these were in part causing her blocked nose. She was sceptical about this, as she had changed her pillow some time before to a polyester one without any obvious benefit. I immediately tested polyester and found that she was sensitive to this as well. A case of out of the frying pan into the fire.

Once when testing a small child I found him allergic to milk and oranges. When I suggested to his mother that this might be aggravating his eczema, she assured me I must be wrong, as she had tried excluding these things to no avail. I asked her if she had excluded them both at the same time. She then realised that when she had excluded milk she had given her child orange juice to drink, and when she had excluded orange juice he had had extra milk.

Cytotoxic Testing

In this test white blood cells from the patient are mixed with the suspected allergen. If the person has an allergy to the substance, the white blood cells begin to degenerate. While this cannot be seen with the naked eye, it can be seen with a microscope by a trained technician.

Substances causing visible cell changes are then identified as allergens. This procedure is solely concerned with IgG4 antibodies. A lot of false-negatives and false-positives may be found using this method, partly because it is a very boring but exacting job for the laboratory technicians involved. There have been a lot of criticisms of its accuracy.

Electroacupuncture According to Voll (EAV) Testing

This procedure was developed by Dr. Reinhold Voll of Germany. The technique utilises an ohmmeter, a hand held probe and a point probe and is designed to measure the skin's electrical activity at designated acupuncture points.

The client holds the negative hand probe in one hand and the practitioner applies the other probe to points on the opposite hand or foot. The application of the probe elicits a very low constant voltage to the acupuncture point being tested. A reading of the residual current flowing through the hand into the ohmmeter is then taken. This can give information on the state of health of various organs and systems of the body. When testing substances for allergies, the test substance is placed onto a testing plate and the point reading is done as normal. The subsequent reading on the ohmmeter would indicate whether or not the person was allergic to that substance. Modern forms of EAV utilise computer software to enhance the effectiveness of the equipment and are now referred to as computerised electro dermal screening devices or 'CEDS devices'. Different models are available from different manufacturers (e.g. Vega, Mora, BEST, Orion, Avatar and QXCI).

ELISA (Enzyme Linked Immunosorbant Assay) Testing

This method is carried out in a laboratory on a pinprick of blood, which can often be sent through the post. The sample is diluted and placed on a plate with various food antigens located in wells. After several procedures, the plate is checked by computer to see if food antibodies have bound to the antigens. This procedure considers IgG 1,2,3 and 4. Only looks at foods. Available by mail order.

Intradermal Skin Testing

This is always carried out in a medical setting. Solutions of allergens are tested by injecting under the skin, and the resulting weal is measured. Increase in weal size denotes an allergen. Sometimes different dilutions are used until a dilution is found which does not produce a weal. This dilution is then given as oral drops or injections to turn off the allergic reaction. A costly, painstaking and painful procedure.

Kinesiology Testing

A system based on manually testing muscle reactions is used to identify allergies. The substance (or a homeopathic/radionic version) is placed either in the mouth or on the body, and the response of one or more muscles is assessed. This allows a whole range of substances to be rapidly checked. There are different branches of kinesiology, some (such as health kinesiology) have a greater interest in allergy problems than others. It can be extremely accurate, but does depend heavily on the knowledge and skill of the practitioner.

Patch Testing

This is usually used for testing for contact allergens, and is carried out in a medical setting. A strip of adhesive with various samples attached to it is placed on the patient's back for 48 hours. When the strip is removed, any raised, reddened or blistered areas are noted and the corresponding substance is regarded as an allergen for that person. A limited range of substances can be tested in this way. Only testing the skin's reaction to substances, so may be misleading.

Pulse Testing

This technique is set out in 'The Pulse Test' by Arthur F. Coca. It is based on the finding that eating allergenic substances causes an increase in the pulse. The pulse is taken at regular intervals before and after meals, on waking and on going to bed. The normal range for the pulse is established, and then individual food items are tested and a pulse reading is taken. Inhalant/contact allergens can sometimes be found this way too. People using this approach often get very anxious, so that the pulse keeps on going up and down independent of anything they are eating, leading to confusing results. Smoking is not allowed during the process. This does not work well if the person has a lot of allergies, particularly to substances in the environment, because exposure to one of these can increase the pulse, while an innocent food is being tested.

Radionic Testing

Radionic practitioners usually use a 'witness' of the client – often a hair sample. They use dowsing to establish problem substances. Very dependent on the skill and knowledge of the individual practitioner.

RAST Testing

RAST stands for Radio Allergo-Sorbent Test. Allergens are mixed with the person's blood. If specific antibodies for that allergen are present in the blood, they will attach themselves to the allergen. Anti-human IgE, tagged with a radioactive label, is added and allowed to combine with the antigen-specific IgE. The level of radioactivity of the sample is measured. This then can be translated into the level of antibody activity in relation to a particular substance. This is looking at only one type of reaction (IgE). Some people who have a lot of allergies have very high levels of total IgE, and this can confuse the test result.

Skin Prick Testing (SPT)

A drop of the suspected allergen is placed on the skin, usually the forearm, and a small prick is made through the drop into the skin, and the reaction is then monitored. If a weal or reddening of the skin occurs, this suggests that the person is allergic to the substance. Unfortunately some people react severely to this form of testing, and children can become quite frightened and unco-operative. Only testing reaction of skin to allergen, so may give inaccurate results.

Scratch Testing

This is a less severe version of the prick test. A drop of the suspected allergen in solution is placed on the skin and then the skin is scratched so that the allergen can enter into the skin. Only testing reaction of skin to allergen, so may be misleading.

Correcting Allergies

It is still widely believed that the only way of addressing allergies is avoidance, but my experience is that this is often unsuccessful.

Once the first flush of enthusiasm has died down, it can be difficult to maintain a diet that avoids some staple (or favourite) food. More importantly, where people are excluding a lot of foods, their diets may become more and more unbalanced. This then makes it likely that they will become allergic to more things, partly because they are eating a limited range of things excessively, and partly because their diet may have become deficient in some important nutrient or nutrients.

There is also a further problem in that if an allergen is avoided, any ability to cope with it may be lost. If this happens, the person is likely to react severely if an accidental encounter with the allergen happens.

Even if it is possible and advisable to avoid foods that are a problem, other substances, such as moulds and pollens, are difficult or even impossible to avoid.

It is fortunate then that there are some effective and pain-free ways of eliminating allergies/intolerances. There are two methods that I particularly recommend, because I have extensive professional experience of them. This is not to say that other methods are not effective.

Kinesiology

Kinesiology and Touch For Health come originally from chiropractic, but have developed to include work with psychological problems, allergies and more. Different branches of kinesiology tackle allergies in different ways.

Health Kinesiology was developed by Jimmy Scott, Ph.D. It includes particularly simple, but highly effective ways of testing for and correcting allergies/intolerances. A short allergy manual can be downloaded from the international web site of health kinesiology:

http://www.subtlenergy.com

This explains how to use muscle testing and acupuncture point balancing quickly and effectively to identify and correct allergy problems. If you are already familiar with basic muscle testing or have some other method for testing for allergies, my book 'Energy Mismatch' teaches the same simple correction procedure, based on the health kinesiology system. This book also extends the concept of allergy to include problems with viruses, hormones, etc.

For more information on health kinesiology contact:

> Health Kinesiology Inc
> Birdsalls House
> RR3 Hastings
> Ontario
> KOL 1YO
> Canada
> Tel: 705 696 3176
> Fax: 705 696 3664
> www.subtlenergy.com
> or

Ann Parker
44 Woodland Way, Old Tupton
Chesterfield
Derbyshire
S42 6JA
Tel: 01246 862339
www.hk4health.co.uk

Isopathic (Homeopathic) Desensitization

Isopathic desensitisation involves giving the client a homeopathic version of the substance to which they react. So, for example, if the client were allergic to apple, they would take a homeopathic dilution of apple over a short period. This approach has been pioneered in the UK by the British Institute For Allergy and Environmental Therapy:

The British Institute for Allergy & Environmental Therapy
Ffynnonwen Pharmacy
Llangwyryfon
Aberystwyth
Mid Wales
SY23 4LY
Tel: 01974 241376
Fax: 01974 241795
allergy@onetel.net.uk
www.allergy.org.uk

Allergens A To Z

In the following pages I am only concerned with looking at these substances from an allergy perspective, not a toxic perspective. It is undoubtedly true, however, that if a person is allergic to a substance, he/she is likely to have more problems counteracting its toxic qualities.

This information should be taken as a guide only. Because an item appears on a list, it does not mean that it will <u>always</u> contain that ingredient, nor are the lists totally comprehensive.

In general, particular substances are not linked to particular symptoms, so cheese could cause *eczema* in one person and *irritable bowel syndrome* or *migraines* in another. I have treated a mother and daughter who both suffered from migraines, but their allergies were completely different.

Although some products are labelled as hypoallergenic, this does not mean that they cannot produce an allergic reaction in a susceptible person. In practice people can be allergic to anything.

One asthmatic child I tested was allergic to non-biological washing powders, and fine on biological ones; another child with *eczema* was allergic to cotton but had no problem with synthetic material. These sorts of situations are not common, but they do alert us to be aware that we should not categorise anything as always safe or always harmful.

There are no 'safe' foods. One of my sons was allergic to carrots, including organic carrots. They made him hyperactive.

Sadly it is impossible to give any guidance about how soon
symptoms appear after contact with an allergen, because the
individual variations are so wide.

A

Abietic Acid
Used extensively in manufacture of *plastics*, *paints*, *varnishes* and
detergents. A by-product of the wood pulp industry.

Acacia Gum
See *gum acacia*.

Accidental Contaminants
When food is processed commercially it may be contaminated with
hydraulic oils, gear oils, air compressor and other lubricants, low
and high temperature application greases, silicone grease and
conveyor and chain lubricants. These will not be listed on the
ingredients. See also *carry over ingredients*.

Acesulfame-K
Also known as E950 and acesulfame potassium. An artificial
sweetener sold commercially as Sunette or Sweet One. Found as a
sugar substitute in packet or tablet form. Also used in *chewing gum*,
dry mixes for beverages, *soft drinks*, non-dairy *creamers*, desserts
and baked goods, particularly when sold as 'sugar-free; or 'low-
calorie'.

Acetaldehyde

Also known as ethanal (not ethanol). Used in the
production of *perfumes*, *polyester resins*, and basic
dyes. Also used as a *solvent* in the *rubber*, *leather*
tanning, and *paper* industries, as a fruit and fish

preservative, as a flavouring agent and for hardening *gelatine*. Added to industrial *alcohol* to discourage consumption of it.

Acetamide MEA
Found in hair preparations including conditioners, *hair dyes* and hair sprays.

Acetate
See *cellulose acetate*.

Acetic Acid
Also known as E260. Used to regulate acidity in food. Typically, *vinegar* is about 4 to 8% acetic acid. Found in chutney, pate, cakes, cough tincture, rheumatic liniment, antiseptic skin applications, wart and corn ointment, hair removal creams, *fungicides*, floor cleaners, and *silicone* sealants. May be sprayed on to silage to discourage bacterial and fungal growth. Also occurs naturally in plant and animal tissues and is involved in fatty acid and carbohydrate metabolism. Produced in the human body after the consumption of alcohol.

Acetic Anhydride
Mainly used in the manufacture of *cellulose acetate* for films and plastic goods, but also used in the synthesis of *aspirin*, the manufacture of industrial chemicals, pharmaceuticals, *perfumes*, *plastics*, synthetic fibres, explosives, and weed killers.

Acetone
Also called dimethyl ketone, 2-propanone, and beta-ketopropane. Found in volcanic gases, forest fires, *vehicle exhaust fumes*, *tobacco smoke*, and landfill sites. Used in *nail polish removers*, many *perfumes*, *paints*, *varnishes*, *solvents*, and cleaning fluids. Also produced in the body primarily during excessive fat metabolism, although some levels present in virtually every organ and tissue, and in the blood.

Acetyl Tributyl Citrate
Found in *nail polish*.

Acrilan
See *acrylic*.

Acrylates Copolymer
Used in *nail polish* and artificial nails.

Acrylamide

 A chemical used in synthetic fibres and waste treatment. Also produced when carbohydrate is baked or fried at high temperatures. Because of health concerns, packaging in Germany now recommends that potato chips are deep fried at a lower temperature for longer.

Acrylic
Also known by the trade names Acrilan, Courtelle and Dralon. Used to make clothing, *carpets* and other household furnishings. Also used as a replacement for asbestos, and reinforcement for *concrete* and stucco, and in some *paints* and *varnishes*.

Adhesives
Can be either derived naturally or made synthetically. Natural adhesives from hide, bones, skin and connective tissues of animals, or from tree gums and plant starches. Synthetic adhesives from *resorcinol*, *epoxy resins*, *methanol*, *hexane*, *heptane* and *toluene*. Waterproof adhesives normally include *silicones*. Widely used in manufacturing. Adhesive on stamps and envelopes is usually *gum Arabic*, *gum tragacanth* or *tapioca* starch. Urea-*formaldehyde* glue used in chipboard manufacture. May also contain chemicals (e.g. *diethylene glycol*) to stop them drying out.

Adipic Acid

A chemical used in the manufacture of *nylon, polyester, polyurethane, polypropylene* and *PVC*. Also used in *detergents*.

Aerosol Propellants

Propane, butane, dimethyl ether and *isobutane* are used in most household aerosol products and air fresheners. Compressed air, carbon dioxide and nitrogen also used in a limited way.

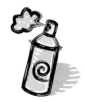

Aflatoxin

A toxin produced by the *mould Aspergillus flavus*, which may be found on *peanuts*, and occasionally also on *grain*, particularly when the crop has been grown under drought conditions.

Agar

Also known as agar-agar, dai choy goh, Japanese isinglass, and kanten. Made from a combination of algaes from the species Gelidium. Used as a gelling agent, thickener and *stabiliser* in foods, as a *tabletting agent*, and as a laxative. Used in seaweed salad served at sushi restaurants.

AHAs

See *alpha-hydroxy acids*.

Air Conditioning Systems

Moulds like the conditions prevalent within air conditioning systems – moist warm air is ideal for them. The problem is not just in homes and work places, a study of car/automobile air conditioning systems showed most contained moulds.

Air Fresheners

Air fresheners work in one of four ways: by interfering with the ability to smell by way of a nerve-deadening agent; by coating nasal passages with a fine oil film; by covering up one smell with another; and (rarely) by breaking down the offensive odour. Generally contain a mixture of different chemicals including *formaldehyde*, and also *perfume*.

Air Pollution

See *pollution*.

Albumen

Another name for egg white. See *egg*.

Alcohol

Also known as ethyl alcohol or ethanol. Found in after-shave lotions, *perfumes*, hand lotions, *nail polishes* and other personal care products, as well as alcoholic drinks. Used as a starting point in the manufacture of other chemicals, and is also used as an industrial *solvent*.

Alginic Acid

Also known as E400. A *stabiliser* commonly used in *ice cream*, cheese, milk shakes, salad dressings, coating for fish and meat, fruit juice, foam on beer, medicines and dressing on textiles.

Allantoin

In *perfume* and some personal care products.

Allspice

Also called Jamaican pepper or pimento. Used in marinades and pickles, and in jars of commercial pickled herrings.

Allura Red AC
An orange-red *food colouring* also known as E129 and FD & C Red 40. Found in confectionary, desserts, drinks, condiments, *drugs* and *cosmetics*. Used extensively in the USA as a replacement for *amaranth*, which is banned. Allura red AC is banned in Denmark, Belgium, France, Germany, Switzerland, Sweden, Austria, Norway, Australia, New Zealand, and Japan.

Aloe Vera
A plant extract, found in personal care products, such as after-sun lotions, deodorants, toning lotions and eye gels. Sometimes used in toilet paper and tissues. Also used as a *nutritional supplement.*

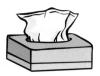

Alpha-Hydroxy Acids
Also known as AHAs. Include *glycolic acid*, *ascorbic acid* and *lactic acid*. Found in many skin care products as exfoliants and moisturisers.

Alternaria
A widespread airborne *mould* occurring both indoors and out. Particularly abundant in decaying plant matter, indoor horizontal surfaces and window frames. A common allergen.

Alum
See *aluminium sulphate.*

Aluminium
A relatively common allergen. Common sources are bleached flour, aluminium cooking pans, aluminium foil and aluminium cans, particularly when the contents are drunk past their sell-by date. Also licensed as a food colouring, E173, but only for external decoration. Some *anti-caking agents* are aluminium based, (e.g. *aluminium silicate*), and these can be found in salt and *baking powder*, and as

carry over ingredients in processed foods. Many deodorants and antacid preparations are also aluminium based. Some *coins* contain aluminium.

Aluminium Hydroxide
Also known as aluminium trihydrate and aluminium hydrate. Used in *vaccines*, manufacture of glass and glazes, as a flame retardant in *plastics*, in *paper* manufacture, printing inks, *detergents*, for waterproofing fabrics, in mouthwashes and deodorants. Also used as a carrier of artificial *colourings* particular for uses involving colouring oils and fats, or where the product does not contain sufficient water to dissolve the colour. (Would not need to be shown in the list of ingredients when used as a colour carrier.)

Aluminium Silicate
Used in medicinal *tablets*, in *rubber* goods, *insecticides*, fire proof blankets, paper and *toothpastes*. Also used in the manufacture of *paints* and printing inks, as an alternative to *titanium dioxide.*

Aluminium Sulphate
Spelt as aluminum sulfate in some countries. Used in pulp and *paper* production, and in the *water* and waste treatment industries.

Aluminum
See *aluminium.*

Aluminum Sulfate
See *aluminium sulphate.*

Amalgam
See *dental amalgam.*

Amaranth

A *food colouring* also known as E123 and FD & C Red 2, Food Red 9 and C.I. 16185. Gives a purplish-red colour, and is found in *ice creams*, gravy granules, soups, jams, jelly, and desserts. Banned in Norway, United States, Russia, Austria, Australia and New Zealand. Allowed in France and Italy only for caviar. There is also a plant known as amaranth, whose leaves and seeds are edible. Used as a flour for those who are avoiding *wheat* or *gluten*. In Mexico used to make alegria (confectionery) and atole (a drink). In Peru used to make a beer, and in both countries boiled and fried as a vegetable. In India used in some confectionery.

Amaretto

A liqueur made from apricot pits, with an almond flavour.

Amines

May form *nitrosamines* under certain circumstances. Compounds that contain amines include *DEA, MEA* and *TEA*.

Ammonia

A chemical found in household cleaners, paint stripper, disinfectants, deodorants, hair bleaches, permanent wave solutions and rheumatic liniments. Used in the manufacture of fertilisers, *plastics* and *nylon*.
Low levels of ammonia are also found in *water*. Sometimes water authorities will deliberately add this as well as *chlorine* where they have been repairing and/or upgrading the mains. Also a metabolic by-product in the body.

Ammonia Lauryl Sulphate

Derived from *coconut*. Used in *cosmetics*, and rug and upholstery shampoos. Mixed with herbicides to ensure optimal coverage of fruit and vegetables, so traces will remain in small amounts on the product in the shops.

Ammonium Hydroxide
Found in hair lightening creams, industrial *solvents* and cleaners.

Ammonium Thioglycolate
Used in permanent wave treatment for hair and also in hair straightening preparations.

Amylcinnamaldehyde
A commonly used synthetic *perfume* present in a wide range of personal care and household products.

Anaesthetics
The main general anaesthetics are desflurane, droperidol, enflurane, etomidate, halothane, isoflurane, ketamine, methohexital, methoxyflurane, midazolam, nitrous oxide, propofol, sevoflurane and thiopental. Several different anaesthetics may be used together. The main local anaesthetics used in dentistry and 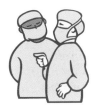 minor surgery are: lignocaine (the most widely used), bupivacaine, mepivacaine, prilocaine, procaine, chloroprocaine and tetracaine. Both local and general anaesthetics can cause sensitivity problems. Many people do not make the connection, but attribute the symptoms to the operation itself. Common symptoms include *nausea*, *tiredness* and *depression*.

Angora
Angora wool comes from the angora rabbit, and is used in clothing. Sometimes the term is also used to refer to wool from the angora goat.

Animal hair
Cat and dog hair remains airborne after it has been disturbed for much longer than *house dust mite*. This is because the particle size is smaller. See also *cat*, *dog* and *rabbit*.

Annatto

A red *food colouring* that comes from the seeds of the annatto tree. Also known as E160(b).Used in *cheese* (e.g. Double Gloucester and Red Leicester cheese), *margarine*, desserts, and some *cosmetics*. Not approved in Australia and New Zealand.

Anthocyanins

Also known as E163. A natural red/blue *food colouring* that comes from black *grapes*, blackcurrants, cherries, elderberries, red cabbage or strawberries. Used in drinks, jams, desserts and confectionary. Also used in *nutritional supplements* for its antioxidant properties.

Antibiotics

Many people react badly to antibiotics. As well as the drug itself, *tabletting agents* and *colourings* may be a problem. See also *penicillin*.

Anti-Caking Agents

Substances that are added to powdered foods such as *salt*, icing sugar and powdered milk to help them to flow more easily. Also used in commercial food preparation. Common ones are various forms of calcium phosphate (also known as E341), calcium silicate, magnesium phosphate (also known as E343), *sodium hexacyanoferrate (II)* and *potassium hexacyanoferrate (II)*. These will not necessarily be declared on the label.

Antimony

Found in solder and *pewter*.

Antioxidants

Added to food to prevent discolouration or rancidity. May be from natural sources or made synthetically. Substances that are used include *ascorbic acid*, calcium ascorbate, *vitamin E, butylated hydroxyanisole*, etc.

Apple

 Individuals allergic to apple may also be allergic to carrot as they share some of the same chemicals, even though they are not in the same botanical family. Used to make *pectin*.

Aqua

Another name for *water*, often used in labelling of *cosmetics* and personal care products. In these circumstances the water is usually purified in some way.

Arachis Oil

A refined preparation of *peanut* oil that does not contain peanut proteins. Used in skin creams and ointments. Thought to be less allergenic, because it does not contain peanut proteins, but a study of children born in the 1990's, which was published in the 'New England Journal of Medicine', found that children who were treated as babies with creams containing peanut oil were nearly seven times more likely to develop a peanut allergy than those who were not. Because of this problem many manufacturers are now using alternatives such as *paraffin*.

Aromatic Compounds

See *phenolic food compounds*.

Arsenic

An ingredient in pigments and wood preservatives. Used as a poison in *pesticides* and herbicides. May also be present in drinking water in areas where there are arsenic deposits in ground.

Artificial Silk

See *rayon*.

Artificial Sweeteners

See *Acesulfame-K, aspartame, mannitol* and *saccharin*.

Asbestos

From fibrous variety of the mineral silica. Found in many products in the home such as roofing and flooring materials, wall and pipe insulation, fireproofing, fireproof clothes, acoustic insulation, some *cements*, coating materials, floor tiles, heating equipment, brake and clutch linings, ironing board pads and textured *paint*. A study of 3,000 autopsies in a New York City hospital showed that half of the individuals had asbestos particles in their lungs. New use of asbestos has been banned in many countries (e.g. EU in 1999, Chile 2001, Australia in 2003, and South Africa in 2004), although asbestos can still legitimately be found in these countries in older products. Russia is the biggest exporter of asbestos, and Canada is the second.

Ascorbic Acid

Also known as vitamin C, E300 and citric acid. *Aspergilla niger* is used in its manufacture. An *antioxidant* and acidity regulator found in food (e.g. instant potato, mustard, tinned meats, *bread, soft drinks, margarine*, jams, jellies, desserts and confectionery). Also found in personal care products (e.g. hair conditioner, shampoo, body wash, baby bath, cleanser, foundation, after-shave) and pharmaceuticals (e.g. cough mixtures) and *nutritional supplements*. Some is also used as *plasticisers* in industry.

Aspartame

Also known as E951. A calorie-free sweetening agent, commonly found in *soft drinks* and low-calorie foods.

Aspergillus Fumigatus

A fungus found in soil and dust and decaying vegetable matter. Particular prevalent in damp straw, compost heaps and birdcages. See *aspergillosis*, page 19.

Aspergillus Glaucus

Common outdoor winter *mould*. Also found on leather.

Aspergillus Niger

A fungus found in soil, dust and decaying vegetable matter. Causes black mould on foodstuffs. Also used in the production of some food additives, e.g.propyl gallate (E310), *octyl gallate* (E311), dodecyl gallate (E312) and *ascorbic acid* (E330).

Asphalt

A mixture of *bitumen* and stones used for road surfaces. In some countries (e.g. the USA) the word 'asphalt' is commonly used to refer to the bitumen on its own.

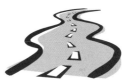

Aspirin

A very common allergen. Individuals who react to aspirin may also react to aspirin-like drugs in painkillers, arthritic drugs and cold remedies. Many people who are allergic to aspirin also react to *azo dyes*. Aspirin originally extracted from willow bark, but now made synthetically. See also *salicylate*.

Astaxanthin

Used in feed for farmed salmon and trout to give a pink pigment to the flesh.

Astra

See *polypropylene*.

Avobenzone
Used in *sunscreen preparations*.

Azodicarbonamide
Also known as azobisformamide. May be added to flour used for *baked goods*.

Azobisformamide
See *azodicarbonamide*.

Azo Dyes
A group of synthetic dyes that all have similar chemical structures. Used in fabrics such as wool and cotton, and in food as they give bright strong colours. *Tartrazine*, yellow 2G, *sunset yellow*, *carmoisine*, *amaranth*, *ponceau 4R*, *red 2G*, brown FK, chocolate brown HT, *black PN* and pigment rubines are azo food dyes. Common allergens.

Azorubine
See *carmoisine*.

B

Bacon
Made from *pork*, which is cured either wet, by immersion in strongly salted water, or dry, by having plain salt or a mix of salt, sugar and spices rubbed in over a period of days. It may also be smoked. *Sodium nitrate* and *sodium nitrite* are often used as preservatives.

Baked Goods
These include cakes, biscuits/cookies and pies. The main ingredients are *flour*, *sugar* and fat.

Eggs are sometimes also used. Biscuits/cookies and pastries are usually made using either plain flour, or plain flour with a little *baking powder* added. Cakes are usually made with self-raising flour. Doughnuts and croissants use *baker's yeast* rather than baking powder. Many other ingredients may also be used, particularly in commercially produced products, e.g. *flavourings, colourings, butylated hydroxyanisole, sodium caseinate, sorbitan monostearate, azodicarbonamide, polyglycerol esters of fatty acids* and *potassium sorbate*.

Baker's Yeast

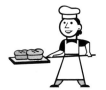

Found in *bread* and in breadcrumbs used to coat savoury and sweet goods. Also used to make doughnuts, but most other *baked goods* use *baking powder* instead. See also *yeast*.

Baking Powder

Consists of *sodium bicarbonate*, one or more acid salts (*cream of tartar* and *sodium aluminium sulphate*) plus *corn* starch to absorb any moisture so a reaction does not take place until a liquid is added. Found in *baked goods*. Added to *flour* to make self-raising flour.

Baking Soda

See *sodium bicarbonate*.

Balsam Of Peru

A *flavouring* used in tobacco, drinks and food, and a *fixative* and fragrance in *perfumes*.

Banana

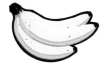

Plantain is the only other member of this botanical family that is eaten.

Bank Notes
Usually made from cotton and *linen*. The ink is applied under extremely high pressure. Various fibres and metal foils are also used to make counterfeiting more difficult.

Barley
Used to make *beer* and *whisk(e)y*. Also found in some coffee substitutes. *Malt* is usually made from barley.

Bauxite
An *aluminium* ore used in road surfacing.

Beds & Bedding
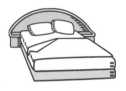
We come into close contact with a lot of different substances while we sleep. Bed may be made from wood and metal. *Mattresses* and pillows can be made from a variety of materials. Duvets/quilts are usually made from *feathers* or *polyester*. Sheets are usually made from *polyester* and/or cotton. *House dust mite* and *detergents* may also be a problem. May be a problem because it's a favourite sleeping spot during the day for a *pet*. See also *mattresses* and *pillows*.

Beer

Made from *brewer's yeast*, malted *barley*, *sugar*, hops and water, although some German and Belgium beers are based on *wheat*. Alcohol free beers are brewed at 1 deg C, a temperature that stops the ingredients fermenting to create alcohol. May also be other ingredients to stabilise foam (e.g. *sodium alginate*).

Bee Sting
A common allergen, which may cause *anaphylactic shock* (see page 18).

Beeswax
A natural product taken from the bee honeycomb. May be found in *mascaras*, lip liners and *lipsticks*, *drugs*, floor and furniture waxes, *shoe polishes* and leather treatments.

Beetroot
In the same food family as beet *sugar*. A *food colouring*, *betanin*, is extracted from it.

Beetroot Red
See *betanin*.

Beet Sugar
See *sugar*.

Bentonite
A kind of clay used in fining *wine* (improving clarity). Also used in the oil drilling industry, cat litter, cosmetics and skin care preparations.

Benzaldehyde
Many synthetic *perfumes* are derived from this chemical.

Benzalkonium Chloride
Antibacterial so used in hand scrubs and face washes. Preservative for drugs and in ophthalmic solutions.

Benzene
Found in *tobacco smoke*, synthetic fibres, *plastics* and *rubbers*, varnishes, lacquers, paint and varnish removers, inks, oils, *detergents* and *pesticides*. Also given off from *petrol*. A survey in 1999 found that British standards are regularly exceeded in urban streets, particularly around petrol stations ('Times' March 2nd 1999).

Benzoic Acid
A food preservative, also known as E210 and butyl paraben. Commonly found in jam, beer, salad cream, *margarine*, *cosmetics*, personal care products, many cough medicines and anti-fungal ointments. Also involved in the manufacture of the preservatives *sodium benzoate* and *potassium benzoate*. Used in the production of caprolactam (for *nylon* fibres).

Benzopyrene
Found in *tobacco smoke*.

Benzoyl Peroxide
An active ingredient in anti-acne preparations.

Benzyl Acetate
Widely used in *perfumed* products to give a 'floral smell'.

Benzyl Alcohol
Also known as phenylmethanol. A component in many naturally occurring *perfume* oils, including jasmine, hyacinth, and ylang-ylang. Used in manufacture of synthetic perfumes and *flavourings*. Found in cosmetics, personal care products and in ointments. Also used as a photographic developer for colour film, as an embedding material in microscopy, and as an industrial *solvent*. Used as a preservative for injectable *drugs*, and in contact lens cleaners.

Beryllium
There may be low levels in some *dental* alloys. Also used in light, structural materials and in nuclear reactors. Although it is sometimes difficult to understand how people are exposed to this metal, I have found in my practice that a surprising number of people are allergic to it and benefit from having this corrected.

Beta Carotene

Also known as E160a. Naturally present in carrots, apricots, canteloupe melon, parsley, spinach, kale and sweet potatoes. Can be converted by the body into vitamin A. Extracted commercially from carrots (using chemical *solvents* such as *hexane*) or produced synthetically. Used as a *colouring* in tinned soup, *soft drinks*, salad cream, mayonnaise, *ice cream*, butter, *margarine*, and *cosmetics*.

Betanin

Also known as E162. A pink/purple *food colouring* made from *beetroot*. Mainly used for frozen, dried, and short shelf-life products, such as *ice creams* and yoghurt.

BHA

See *butylated hydroxyanisole*.

BHT

See *butylated hydroxytoluene*.

Birch Pollen

Individuals who are sensitive to birch pollen may also react to *apple*, cherries, spinach and *carrot*, as they share some of the same chemicals. *Xylitol* is made from birch.

Biscuits

See *baked goods*.

Bismarck Brown

Also known as Basic Brown 1, and C.I. 21000. Used to *dye* wool and cotton and in *hair dye* preparations. Use is becoming less common.

Bismuth

Found in lead-free solder.

Bismuth Citrate
Used in *hair dyes*.

Bisphenol A
A major constituent of *epoxy resins* and *polycarbonate*. Also used as a sealant and in *adhesives* including in dentistry.

Bitumen
Found in damp proof courses, flat roofs, road surfacing, rust treatment, sealant, carpet tile backing and *pesticides*. Also see *asphalt*.

Black PN
A *food colouring* also known as E151, brilliant black PN and C.I. 28440. Used in fish paste, savoury snacks, mustard, sauces, soups, red fruit jams, flavoured milk drinks, *soft drinks*, desserts, *ice cream* and confectionery. Banned in Denmark, Australia, Austria, Belgium, Canada, Finland, France, Germany, Japan, Norway, Switzerland, Sweden and USA.

Bleach
May be chlorine or peroxide based. See *hydrogen peroxide*, sodium hypochlorite and sodium hydroxide.

Botanical Food Families
See appendix 2.

Bottled Gas
This is *propane* or *butane*.

Bottled Water
Does not necessarily originate from a spring; can be taken from the municipal *water* supply. Most bottlers use ozone gas to disinfect the water instead of *chlorine*. *Plastic* bottles may be made of *polyethylene terephthalate*, high-density *polyethylene* or *polycarbonate*.

Contaminants of concern in bottled water include arsenic, bacteria, parasites, and synthetic chemicals such as *phthalates*.

Bourbon

In order for a drink to be called 'bourbon' more than 50 percent of the grain used must be *corn*, and it must be aged for a minimum of two years in charred oak barrels.

Boysenberry

A hybrid of loganberry, raspberry and blackberry.

Brandy

Made from *grapes* and *brewer's yeast*. Sometimes aged in oak casks. Also used to fortify *sherry*.

Brass

An alloy of *copper* and *zinc*. Used for some *coins*, door and furniture fittings, and in model toy making.

Bread

Main ingredients are *grain* (predominantly *wheat* and *rye*) and *baker's yeast*. Flour improvers such as *ascorbic acid* often added. *Sodium stearoyl lactylate* and *sodium stearyl fumarate* used as dough strengtheners. Malted *barley* used in granary bread. See also *toast*.

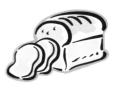

Breast Milk

Babies can be allergic to breast milk, but it is usually proteins that have travelled into the breast milk from food eaten by the mother or else chemical contaminants. The World Wide Fund for Nature (WWF) says more than 350 man-made pollutants have been identified in the breast milk of women in the UK. One of my sons suffered from projectile vomiting as a small baby, but only if I had eaten *eggs*. The vomiting would occur when I breast-fed him about

8 hours after I had eaten the eggs. Testing showed he was allergic to eggs.

Brewer's Yeast
Used to make *alcohol*, *vinegar* and *yeast extract*. Also used in some *nutritional supplements* containing B vitamins.

Brilliant Black PN
See *black PN*.

Brilliant Blue FCF
A bright blue *food colouring* also known as E133, FD & C Blue No 1 and C.I. 42090. Commonly found in confectionery, condiments, icing/frosting, *soft drinks* and tinned peas. Often used with *tartrazine* to give a green colour. Banned in Austria, Belgium, Denmark, France, Germany, Greece, Italy, Norway, Spain, Sweden and Switzerland.

Bromine
A chemical used in the manufacture of *fumigants*, flameproofing agents, disinfectants and photographic materials. May also be found in *swimming pool water* as an alternative to *chlorine*, although not widely used.

Bromodichloromethane
A *trihalomethane*, also known as BDCM. Found in drinking *water* and *swimming pool water* when *chlorine* disinfectants combine with naturally occurring organic matter (including skin cells and urine) to produce this chemical.

Bronze
A mixture of *copper* and *tin*. Many modern 'copper' *coins* are made from bronze.

Bubble Gum
See *chewing gum*.

Buckwheat
In spite of its name buckwheat is not related to *wheat*, but is a member of the same family as rhubarb. Can be a useful food for people who are avoiding *gluten* or *grains*.

Bulgar
A form of *wheat*.

Butadiene
See *styrene*.

Butane
A by-product of petroleum refining. Used as a propellant in hair mousses and sprays, as fuel in cigarette lighters, small blowtorches, camping stoves, outdoor portable lanterns and patio heaters.

Buteth-3
Found in *hair dyes* and personal care products.

Butoxyethanol
Used as a *solvent* in *cosmetics* and personal care products.

Butter
Made from *cow's milk*. Allergy to dairy products is often an allergy to a protein in the milk. As butter is fat, some people who are allergic to milk can eat butter without any problem.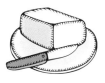

Butyl Acetate
Found in wood fillers, tile adhesives and *nail polishes*.

Butyl Paraben
See *benzoic acid*.

Butyl Rubber
Also known as polyisobutylene (which is the major constituent). A synthetic rubber used for tyre inner tubes, hoses, roofing, pond liners, and in biomedical *joint replacements*. See also *rubber*.

Butylated Hydroxyanisole
Also known as BHA and E320. Probably the most extensively used *antioxidant* for food. Mostly used in foods that are high in fats and oils, such as sausages, mayonnaise and *baked goods*. May also be in confectionary, stock cubes, personal care products, *cosmetics* and *drugs*.

Butylated Hydroxytoluene
An *antioxidant* that is also known as BHT and E321. Typical products include foods containing fats and oils, personal care products, cosmetics, *detergents* and *drugs*. Also incorporated into packaging in, for example, the inner packaging of breakfast cereals.

Butylene Glycol
In after-sun lotions, deodorants, skin toners, moisturisers and other personal care products. Used in the production of *polyester* and *polyurethanes*.

C

Cadmium
A toxic metal found in *tobacco smoke*, nickel-cadmium batteries, galvanised iron, *pesticides*, *plastics*, fertilisers, tyres, plating, colour

TV tubes, *PVC* (as a *stabiliser*), industrial *paints*, artists paints, and pottery. Also a component in alloys and solder. Low levels in all foods (highest in shellfish, liver, and kidney meats).

Caffeine
Found in *coffee*, *tea*, guarana, *soft drinks* (particularly *colas*), sports drinks, *chocolate*, some painkillers and tonics. See also *decaffeination process* and *cola*.

Cakes
See *baked goods*.

Calcium Alginate
Also known as E404. Typically used as a thickener in desserts. Also used in moist wound dressings.

Calcium Carbonate
See *chalk*.

Calcium Chloride

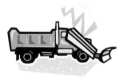

Also known as E509. Used for de-icing roads, and in dust control Also used as an anti-freeze in *concrete* mixes and in refrigeration plants, and as a food preservative.

Calcium Hydroxide
Also known as slaked lime. Used in the production of mortar, in sugar refining and in the production of other chemicals. Used to remove hair from the hides in leather tanning.

Calcium Orthophosphates
See *anti-caking agents*.

Calcium Oxide

Also known as lime. Used in agriculture, and the construction industry. Also used in the manufacture of *steel*, glass, *paper* and *sugar*, and in the treatment of water and sewage.

Calcium Thioglycollate

See *acetic acid*.

Calvados

A *brandy* distilled from *apple* cider, produced only in the French region of Normandy.

Candelilla Wax

Extracted from the plant Euphorbia Cerifera, and used in *cosmetics* (particularly in creams and *lipsticks*).

Candida

See *candidiasis* (page 21).

Cane Sugar

See *sugar*.

Canola Oil

The American name for *rapeseed* oil.

Capsanthin

Also known as E160(c). An orange /red *food colouring* derived from paprika. Used in poultry feed to deepen the colour of egg yolks. Not permitted in Australia and New Zealand.

Capsules

Most capsules are made from *gelatine*. *Plasticisers*, such as *glycerine*, added to soften gelatine capsules. Vegetarian/Kosher/Halal capsules (used for some *nutritional supplements*) made from *hydroxypropyl methylcellulose*. Usually fewer inactive ingredients than *tablets*.

Car Exhaust
See *vehicle exhaust fumes*.

Carageenan
A type of seaweed, also known as Irish moss and E407. Used as a *stabiliser* in salad dressings, processed cheeses, prepared meats and fish, *ice creams*, cakes, *toothpastes* and shaving creams.

Caramel
A *food colouring* also known as E150. Usually manufactured from cane *sugar*. Products that may contain it include brown *bread*, and other *baked goods*, decorations, fillings and toppings, crisps, gravy browning, pickles, sauces and dressings, *soft drinks*, dessert mixes, confectionery, *vinegar*, *beer* and *wines*.

Carbolic Acid
See *phenol*.

Carbomer
Found in hand creams, body lotions, shower gels, hair gels, medicated face washes, after-shave lotions and other personal care products, particularly those that are gel based.

Carbon Black
Also known as acetylene black, channel black, furnace black, lamp black, thermal black, and noir de carbone. Used as a reinforcing agent in *rubber* products such as tyres, conveyor belts, tubes etc. Used as a black pigment in carbon paper, printing, polishes, ink, *photocopier toner*, etc.

Carbon Monoxide
A major air pollutant, mainly from traffic, although catalytic converters and other new technologies have reduced the problem from this source. Also produced by badly vented indoor stoves, fireplaces, candles, incense and *cigarette* smoke.

Carbon Tetrachloride
Has been used in fire extinguishers, as a *dry cleaning* agent, in making *nylon*, as a *solvent* for soaps and insecticides, etc. Banned in some countries because of clear evidence that it is carcinogenic, and use declining elsewhere.

Carboxylate
Used as driers for the printing ink and paint industries, and as a bonding material in dentistry.

Carboxymethyl Cellulose
See *sodium carboxymethyl cellulose*.

Carminic Acid
A red *food colouring* from the Dactilopium coccus insect, also known as carmine of cochineal, E120, C.I. 75470, and natural red 4. Used in food and cosmetic products.

Carmoisine
A *food colouring* also known as E122, azorubine, food red 3 and C.I. 14720. Common uses include confectionery, yoghurts, ices, jams and preserves. Banned in Japan, Norway, Sweden and the United States.

Carnauba Wax
From the South American Copaiba palm. Used in drug *tablets*, confectionery, *mascaras* and other *cosmetics*, deodorants, furniture polishes and *varnishes*.

Carob

A bean from the legume family. Used as an alternative to *chocolate* in products marketed for people with a chocolate allergy. *Locust bean gum* is also derived from it.

Carob Bean Gum

See *locust bean gum*.

Carotenoids

Over 400 carotenoids have been identified. The ones used as *food colourings* come mainly from annatto, *carrots*, oranges, red peppers and tomatoes, and are yellow, orange and red. Listed in Europe as various sub-categories of E160 and E161, e.g. *capsanthin* is E160c. Uses include *margarine*, dairy products and *soft drinks*. See also *beta carotene*.

Carpets

A variety of yarns are used including *nylon*, *polypropylene* (also known by the trade names Olefin, Astra, Zylon and Charisma), *acrylic* (Acrilan, Courtelle and Dralon), *polyester* (Dacron and Trevira), *rayon* and *wool*. Cotton, *rayon*, *nylon*, *rubber latex* or *polyethylene* may be used for backing.
Adhesives and rubber may have been used in their manufacture. A laboratory test of a sample of carpet dust from an average home revealed high levels of *pesticides*, *polychlorinated biphenols*, and metals such as lead, *cadmium* and *mercury* ('Daily Telegraph' 3 May 2001). These were mainly brought into the house on soles of shoes, or paws of pets, or used in cleaning products. *Tobacco smoke*, *house dust mites* and *moulds* were also present. Babies and small children are more at risk from carpets because they touch them more, and are more likely to put their hands in their mouth after touching them.

Carrot

Individuals allergic to carrot may also be allergic to apple as they share some of the same biochemicals. Other foods that are botanically similar and may cause problems include parsley, parsnip, dill, cumin and celery. The food additive *beta carotene* is sometimes extracted from carrots.

Carry Over Ingredients

'Carry over' ingredients do not need to be listed on labels, because they do not serve any technological function in the finished product. For example, *colourings* may be dissolved in a *solvent* so that the colouring can be distributed more uniformly throughout the product. The colouring would be listed in the ingredients for the finished product, but the solvent would not. Anti-caking chemicals may be added to ensure that powders flow more easily and do not clog the machinery. Anti-foaming agents may be present, added to control the amount of foam produced during manufacture. Although these carry over ingredients are present in the finished product only in minute quantities, this may still be enough to cause problems for some people.

Casein

One of the principal proteins found in *milk*, and the main protein in curds. The harder the *cheese* the more casein it contains. Used in food production and *wine* fining. See also *whey*.

Cashmere

Yarn from goat hair, used to make luxury knitted clothing.

Cassava

A tropical plant. Its root is a staple food in some African and Asian countries. *Tapioca* is made from it.

Castor Oil
A natural plant product used medicinally as a mild purgative, and also used to make polyamide/nylon 11 (a plastic used in engineering), lubricating grease, coatings, inks, sealants, aircraft lubricants, surfactants, emulsifiers, encapsulants, plastic films, and components for shatterproof safety glass. Used in *cosmetics* particularly *lipstick*.

Cat
Often the allergy is not to the cat hair itself but to a protein (Felix domesticus I) present in the dander (skin flakes) and saliva. Cats deposit this protein on their fur when they groom themselves. Male cats tend to be more of a problem as they produce more of the protein. Light haired cats tend to be less of a problem. Cat allergen particles are sticky and become attached to walls, *carpets*, curtains, etc. Have been found in public places (including schools) where cats have never been, carried into these areas on the clothes of the cat owners.

Caustic Soda
See *sodium hydroxide*.

Cavity Wall Insulation
Main materials used are mineral wool (spun from rock or glass), urea *formaldehyde* foam or *polystyrene* beads.

Cellophane
Made from *cellulose* and used as a wrapping for foodstuffs and cigarettes, but is now being replaced by other materials.

Cellular Plastics
See *expanded plastics*.

Cellulose
The chief constituents of plant cell walls. Derived commercially mainly from wood pulp and cotton. Used to make *cellulose acetate*, *sodium carboxymethyl cellulose*, and vegetarian *capsules* for nutritional supplements.

Cellulose Acetate
Made from *cellulose* through the action of *acetic anhydride*. Used to make *rayon* and some photographic films. Also used to make handles for tools, spectacle frames (although now moulded plastics generally used) and *cigarette filters*.

Cement
Made from limestone and other materials (e.g. sand, *clay*, shale.)

Ceteareth-20
Used in personal care products, cosmetics and *hair dyes*.

Cetearyl Alcohol
An emulsifying wax from vegetable sources. Used in *cosmetics* and skin care preparations.

Cetyl Alcohol
An emulsifying wax from vegetable sources. Found in *cosmetics* and personal care products (e.g. shampoos, hair conditioners, tanning lotions, deodorants, sports body rubs, cleansers, body lotions, *lipsticks*, skin creams and after-shave lotions), medicinal ointments and creams.

CFCs
See *chlorofluorocarbons*.

Chaetomium
Mould found on wood, paper, natural fibres such as *jute*, and water-damaged walls.

Chalk

Also known as calcium carbonate. The most common exposure to chalk used to be in classrooms, but with the advent of over-head projectors and white boards this is no longer the case. Used in *toothpaste*, and some sports (e.g. in snooker on the end of the cue). Small amounts may be present on new *rubber gloves*.

Charcoal

Produced when wood is burnt slowly with reduced oxygen. Used in barbecue bricks and *water filters*.

Charisma

See *polypropylene*.

Cheese

Hard cheese contains very little *lactose*. Some cheese contains *histamine*. Mature cheese is rich in *tyramine*. The harder the cheese, the more *casein* it contains. See also *rennet*. May contain colouring and moulds.

Chewing Gum

Contains *chicle* and possibly synthetic gum, as well as softeners (e.g. *colophony*), sweeteners (e.g. *sugar*, *corn* syrup, *xylitol* etc.) and *flavourings*. The dusting on some chewing gum is from *mannitol*.

Chicken

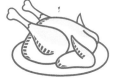 May also be allergic to chicken *eggs*.

Chicle

A resin from a Mexican tree (Achras sapita) used in the manufacture of *chewing gum*.

China Clay
See *kaolin*.

Chinese Insect Wax
Secreted by Coccus ceriferus and used to make candles and polishes.

Chinese Food
Chinese restaurant syndrome (see page 22) is usually attributed to *monosodium glutamate*, but researchers have found that fermented soya and shellfish sauces are likely alternative culprits. (Monosodium glutamate is widely used in Western processed food too.)

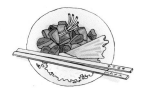

Chloracetamide
A preservative frequently used in *cosmetics*, personal care products and *adhesives*. A common allergen.

Chloramine
Use by some drinking *water* authorities instead of, or as well as, *chlorine*. May be used to help reduce *trihalomethanes* levels in the water. Chloramine also produced when chlorine oxidises dirt in water, so may be found in *swimming pools* and in drinking water. The presence of high levels of chloramines will tend to result in an unpleasant taste and smell to the water.

Chlorine
Found in *bleach*, antiseptics, disinfectants, mould inhibitors, and many *paper* products. One of the basic materials of the chemical industry, used in the production of *solvents*, *vinyl chloride*, refrigerants and *aerosol propellants*. Chlorine washes are used in the processing of prepared salad packs, and some residues will

remain on finished product, and some *chloramine* will also be present. Found in drinking *water* and *swimming pool water*, including where ozone or UV light cleaning systems are in use. A surprising amount of chlorine is inhaled while taking a shower. See also *chloramine* and *swimming pool water*.

Chlorofluorocarbons
Also known as CFCs. A group of chemical compounds containing chlorine, fluorine and carbon. Were used extensively as aerosol propellants and refigerants, but now banned in most countries because of effect on ozone layer. May still be used in *asthma* inhalers.

Chloroform
See *trihalomethanes*.

Chlorophyll
Green *food colourings* also known as E140 and E141, derived commercially from alfalfa and nettles. The chlorophyll is extracted using *acetone*, *ethanol*, light *petroleum*, methylethylketone and diachloromethane. May be found in *chewing gum*, *ice cream*, parsley sauce, soups, confectionery, soap and *drugs*. Also occurs naturally in green vegetables.

Chocolate
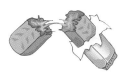 Basic ingredients are cocoa, and *sugar*. Some contains *cow's milk*. In the UK a lot of chocolate contains the artificial flavour *vanillin*. More expensive chocolate usually contains *vanilla*. Other artificial and natural flavours may be included. Cheaper chocolate in the UK and America also generally includes *vegetable fat* (*palm*, coconut, *soya*, cottonseed etc.). White chocolate does not contain any chocolate liquor, but does contain cocoa butter. Chocolate is rich in *tyramine*.

Chromates

Chromium compounds, found in various products, such as *cement*, *leather* tanning, matches, metal plating, *paper* and *paint*. Also found in cleaning solutions in the printing industry, as corrosion inhibitors in open and closed cooling-water systems, in anti-rust paint, wood ash, and ash from burned rubbish.

Chrome

See *chromium*.

Chromium

Used in electroplating, and as an additive for steel to prevent rusting, as an industrial catalyst, and to colour glass emerald green. Chromium is a nutritious mineral, so may be found in some *nutritional supplements*.

Chymosin

Also known as rennin. A milk-clotting enzyme found in the stomach of young mammals, which is used in *cheese* making. Can also be made from micro-organisms by adding genetic information to them so that they produce chymosin.

C.I. Numbers

Colour Index numbers are allocated by the Society of Dyers and Colourists. The index includes information on commercial names, methods of application, etc. for colours used in food, personal care products, *cosmetics*, household products and fabric dyeing. Substances may have both a C.I. number and an *E number*. See appendix 1 for individual C.I. numbers.

Cider

The main ingredients are apples and *brewer's yeast*.

Cigarette Filters

Filters are usually made from *cellulose acetate*, and studies have shown that smokers commonly ingest and/or inhale some of these fibres ('Inhalation Toxicology', 14: 247-262,2002). See also *cigarettes*.

Cigarettes

Smokers may react to the unlit tobacco, the paper and gums used to make the cigarettes, the tobacco *smoke* and/or the *cigarette filters*. Chemicals may also be used to keep the tobacco moist (e.g. *glycerol*).

Cinnamaldehyde

Usually derived from cinnamon bark rather than produced synthetically. Used as a *flavouring*. A common allergen.

Cinnamic Acid

Use as a *flavouring*, and in *perfumes*, *cosmetics* and medicinal products to give a spicy, oriental perfume. Also used to make synthetic *indigo* dye.

Cinnamic Alcohol

Used as a *perfume* and *flavouring*. A common allergen.

Citric Acid

See *ascorbic acid*.

Citronellol

A common artificial *perfume*. Found in personal care products, *cosmetics* and household products.

Citrus Fruit

These include oranges, lemons and grapefruit. Common allergens. Used to make *pectin*.

Citrus Red

A *food colouring*. The US FDA restricts it to specific uses such as colouring orange skins.

Cladosporium Herbarum

One of the most common airborne *moulds* with a world-wide distribution. Common on windowsills, painted walls and *air-conditioning* ducts and similar supply duct. In Europe spores are particularly prevalent in June. A common allergen, often involved in *asthma*.

Clay

The obvious source of this is in pottery, and although it seems relatively inert in this form, some people do still react. Also used extensively as a filler in the manufacture of *paper* and board, as a coating on fertiliser pellets, in some *rubbers* (both synthetic and natural) and *plastics*, in household *paints*, crayons, pencils, *toothpastes* and *cosmetics*. Also see *kaolin*.

Clove Oil

See *eugenol*.

Coal Tar

Thick liquid tar obtained from bituminous coal containing *benzene*, *xylene*, *naphthalene*, *phenol* and *creosol*. Coal tar derivatives include some food additives, *phenol*, *asphalt*, *benzene* and *creosote*. Also used in some *eczema* and psoriasis treatment creams and shampoo. See also *azo dyes*.

Coal Tar Dyes

See *azo dyes*.

Cobalt

Found in *dental* alloys, paper clips, safety pins, watchbands, spectacle frames, *cement*, *tattoos*, pottery dyes, *hair dyes* and lacquers, fly paper, printing ink, watercolour paints and coloured crayons. May also be included in metal prostheses, such as *joint replacements*.

Cobalt Acetylmethionate

Found in antiperspirants and personal care products.

Cocamide DEA

An oil originating from coconut which thickens personal care lotions, e.g. shampoos, bath products, and *cosmetics*. See also *nitrosamines* and *diethanolamine*.

Cocamidopropyl Betaine

Found in shampoos, bubble baths and *liquid soap*.

Cochineal

See *carminic acid*.

Cockroach

 Endemic in some areas. High proportion of *asthma* and *allergic rhinitis* sufferers react to the saliva, faeces and body parts.

Coconut

Several chemicals used in the personal care industry are derived from coconut, e.g. *cocamide DEA*, *lauramide DEA*, *myristyl myristate*. Also may be used to make the carbon in carbon block *water filters*.

Coffee

A common allergen, but sometimes people think they are allergic to coffee (or tea, etc.), but it may be what they put in the drink – *milk*, *sugar* or *artificial sweeteners*. Also used as a flavouring in cakes, chocolates, etc. See also *decaffeination process* and *coffee creamers*.

Coffee Creamer

 Used in *coffee* and *tea* in place of *milk*. Ingredients include *hydrogenated vegetable oils*, *corn* syrup, *maltodextrin*, *sugar*, dipotassium phosphate, and *mono and diglycerides of fatty acids*. Dairy ones often contain *sodium caseinate*.

Coffee Substitutes
These usually contain *grains*, chicory or dandelion root.

Coins
The 'silver' coins used by many countries (e.g. USA, Britain, Australia) are usually made from *cupronickel*. The British one pound and two pound coins are made mainly from *copper*, with some *nickel* and *zinc*. The British one and two pence coins are made from *copper*, *zinc* and *tin*. The US cent is made from *copper*-plated *zinc*. Many Canadian coins are made from *steel* with small amounts of *copper* and *nickel*. Many of the coins of the European Union are made from Nordic gold (89% *copper*, with *aluminium*, *zinc* and *tin*). This is because of concerns about *nickel* allergies. Many years ago I treated a client for arthritis in her hands. She turned out to be allergic to one of the metals used to make fruit machine tokens, and her job involved handling a lot of these every day, as she owned a fruit machine business. Fixing her metal allergy made a significant difference to her hands.

Cointreau
A liqueur made from *brandy* and orange peel.

Cola
Extracted from an African tree. Contains *caffeine*.

Collagen

From animals, usually cows or chickens, but occasionally fish. In plastic surgery may be human collagen. See also *hydrolysed collagen*.

Collagen Replacement Therapy

This form of plastic surgery uses *collagen* from cows or from human sources.

Colophony

Also known as rosin. A pine resin made from *turpentine*. Found in *paper*, cosmetics, *varnishes*, *paint*, polishes, fly-papers, adhesive tapes, depilating waxes, solder flux, etc. Also used as a softener in *chewing gum*.

Colourings

Intensely coloured natural and synthetic compounds used to colour metals, plastics, *fabrics*, *paper*, photography, *paints*, hair, *cosmetics*, personal care products, foods, drinks, etc. Naturally sourced colours may use chemical *solvents* for extraction. Many colours will also contain mineral salts (often *aluminium hydroxide*, but also barium and calcium compounds). As well as the pigment itself there will be carriers, fixatives and *degreasers*. Chemicals involved may include *toluene* and biphenyl butyl benzoate. Food colourings are highly regulated in most countries, so many chemicals are not allowed. See also *food colourings*, *FD & C*, *E numbers*, *C.I. Numbers*, *hair dyes*, and *indigo*.

Combustion

When a substance is burnt during use, new chemicals are produced. People may be allergic to one form but not the other, e.g. *tobacco* rather than *tobacco smoke*. They may be allergic to both, e.g. *petrol*/gas vapours (as experienced while filling a car/automobile) and *vehicle exhaust fumes*.

Condoms

Made from *latex* with the addition of other chemicals, such as accelerators, antioxidants and *dyes*. Most condoms will also have lubricants, spermicides and/or powders. The most frequent powder now used is *corn* starch.

Cookies

See *baked goods*.

Cooking Food

Cooking food changes it in various ways, so it is possible to be sensitive to a food raw and not to it cooked. This most commonly occurs with fruit, vegetables, tuna, *milk* and *eggs*. Occasionally a person is allergic to cooked food and not the raw equivalent, but this is much less common. Overall the most likely situation is that the person will be sensitive to the food in both the raw and the cooked state.

Copper

Used in the manufacture of copper water pipes, wiring, brake linings, *coins*, *drugs*, *pesticides*, *fungicides*, inter-uterine contraceptive devices (copper coil) and *dental amalgam*. Also a component of *brass*, *bronze* and sometimes *pewter*.

Corn

This is *gluten*-free. Found in popcorn, breakfast cereals, *bourbon* and other American *whiskeys*. Also used as a thickener in sauces and other dishes. Corn syrup is used as a sweetener in many manufactured desserts, and as maize starch in tablets. The powder used in the finishing of *condoms* and inside *latex* gloves may be corn starch. See also *glucose* and *dextrose*. Being used to replace talc in personal care and baby products.

Cosmetics

A wide variety of ingredients including oils and waxes (e.g. *lanolin, carnauba wax*, etc.), *colourings* (*titanium dioxide, iron oxide, tartrazine, amaranth*, etc), *perfume* (e.g. *hydroxycitronellal* and *geraniol*), preservatives (e.g. *parabens*, dehydroacetic acid, etc.) and other chemicals (e.g. *glycerol* to keep ingredients moist).

Cotinine

Nicotine is broken down into this in the body. Highly addictive. Can be detected in the blood and urine of children and adults exposed to *tobacco smoke* in their environment, as well as that of smokers. Has been found in the breast milk of smokers. Persists in the system longer than nicotine.

Courtelle

See *acrylic*.

Cow's Milk

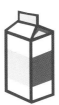
Cow's milk allergy is extremely common. Some of the proteins in cow's milk are affected by heat, and so some individuals who react to these heat-sensitive proteins may be able to tolerate heat-treated milk, e.g. UHT or evaporated milk. See also *lactose*.

Cream Of Tartar

Also known as potassium hydrogen tartrate. Used *in baking powder*.

Crème de Cassis

A blackcurrant liqueur.

Creosote
Distilled from *coal tar*. Used as a wood preservative and disinfectant. A common allergen. People who like the smell of creosote are often allergic to it.

Cresols
Exposure comes from *vehicle exhaust fumes, tobacco smoke* and coal and wood smoke. Cresols occur naturally in oils of various plants (e.g. yucca, jasmine, Easter lily, conifers and oak trees).

Crockery
Usually made from *clay*, with glazes. Although these are seen as being relatively inert, both the clay and the glazes may be a problem for some people.

Crude Oil
This is oil as it comes out of the ground, before processing. The starting material for petrol/gasoline and diesel, and also used to produce many *plastics* and chemicals. Sometimes correcting a crude oil sensitivity will correct an allergy/intolerance to a large range of products.

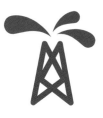

Cupronickel
An alloy of *copper* and *nickel*. Most common material for modern 'silver' *coins*. Also used for marine applications, such as boat propellers.

Curcumin
Also known as E100. A *food colouring* manufactured from *turmeric* using *methanol, hexane* and *acetone*. Typical products include *margarine*, pickles, soup, *ice cream*, desserts and confectionary.

Currants

Small black *grapes* (often Zante or Corinth varieties) that have been dried.

Cutlery

Mainly made from stainless *steel* with handles of *plastic*, wood, or stainless steel. A surprising number of people react to these.

Cyclohexane

Mainly used in the production of *nylon*, but some also used in the production of *solvents*, insecticides and *plasticisers*.

D

Dairy Products

An intolerance to dairy products is not necessarily a *lactose* intolerance. Lactose is a milk sugar, but it is often the milk proteins that cause the problem. Ingredients that contain or may contain dairy include: animal fat, *casein*, *sodium caseinate*, hydrolysed casein, hydrolysed whey, *lactose*, lactalbumin, lactoglobulin, *whey* and *ghee*. See also *cow's milk*, *butter*, *cheese*, *goat's milk* and *sheep's milk*.

D & C

A classification used by the American Food and Drink Administration to categorise *colours* that have been approved for use in drugs and *cosmetics* (but not in food). See also *FD & C*.

Dacron

See *polyester*.

Dander
The tiny particles of skin that are shed by animals such as *cats* and *dogs*. All furry animals shed dander. Long-haired animals do not necessarily produce more dander than short-haired ones.

DBA
See *dibromoacetic acid.*

DEA
See *diethanolamine.*

Deadly Nightshade Family
A botanical group containing *tomato*, *potato*, *tobacco*, chilli, etc. See appendix 2.

Decaffeination
There are three types of decaffeination process used for *tea* and *coffee*. Swiss water process does not involve chemicals and extracts over 90% of the *caffeine*. Usually used for more expensive coffees. Another method involves using a chemical solvent (often includes *methylene chloride* or *ethyl acetate*). This method extracts a higher proportion of caffeine. Highly pressurized carbon dioxide is the third possibility. This removes a high level of caffeine and minimises the detrimental effect of solvent use. Regardless of the decaffeination process used there will always be some caffeine left in the end product.

Degreasers
Chemicals such as *toluene*, *xylene* and citrus oil used to remove grease from a wide range of substances, including wool, plastics and engine parts. Also used in general cleaning products.

Dehydroacetic Acid
A preservative used in personal care products and *cosmetics.*

Denim

Cotton cloth dyed with *indigo*. Pumice stones were traditionally used in the making of indigo denim, but now the enzyme glucanase is more commonly used. *Sodium hypochlorite* may be used to give a faded look to the cloth.

Dental Amalgam

Amalgam is a mixture of metals – over half is *mercury* (in some older fillings that can be nearer three quarters), mixed with *copper*, *tin*, *silver* and *zinc*. Mercury vapour can be released into the mouth from these fillings, although the British Dental Association takes the view that the amount is so low as to be insignificant.

Dental Fillings

May be made from metals (*dental amalgams* or *gold)*, composite *plastic* materials or porcelain.

Dental Treatment

A wide range of different materials and chemicals are used, including metals, *adhesives*, *acrylic*, porcelains, dyes, *anaesthetics*, etc.

Detergents

A complex mixture of chemicals including *sodium carbonate*, *sodium carboxymethyl cellulose* (to stop grime re-attaching to fabric), sodium silicate (to protect the appliance), sodium perborate (bleaching agent), tetra acetyl ethylene diamine (a bleach activator), etc. Biological powders also contain enzymes such as protease, lipase, and amylase. Detergent residues remain even after rinsing, partly because some of the chemicals present are designed to stay in the fabric (e.g. optical brighteners). Sensitivity to detergents is particularly likely in those suffering from skin, nasal and respiratory complaints. Unfortunately it is not possible to recommend particular brands of washing powders, because none of them are safe for everyone. The general rule though is that non-biological powders are likely to be a lesser problem than biological ones. Also used in food processing, and small amounts may remain in finished products.

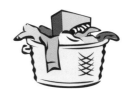

Dextrose
A sweetener usually derived from *corn* (or occasionally from *wheat*), and used in many processed foods. See also *glucose*.

DHA
See *dihydroxyacetone*.

Diammonium Phosphate
Also known as ammonium phosphate and DAP. Used as a yeast nutrient in *wine* making, as a dough strengthener, a fertiliser, a corrosion inhibitor and a flame retardant.

Diazepam
Also known as valium. A minor tranquilliser. Used intravenously as a pre-*anaesthetic* sedative.

Dibromoacetic Acid
Also known as DBA. Found in drinking *water* when *chlorine* disinfectants combine with naturally occurring organic matter.

1, 2-Dichloroethane
See *ethylene dichloride*.

Diesel

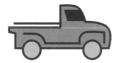

Used for lorries, trucks, trains, buses, some taxis and some cars/automobiles. See *vehicle exhaust fumes*.

Diethanolamine

Used in manufacture of *paper packaging* that will be in contact with food. DEA itself is used in very few *cosmetics*, but DEA-related ingredients (e.g. *cocamide DEA* , *cocamide MEA*, *lauramide DEA* and *TEA-lauryl sulphate*) widely used in personal care products as emulsifiers and foaming agents. Under certain circumstances may produce *nitrosamines*.

Di(2-ethylhexyl) Phthalate

Also known as DEHP. A *plasticiser* added to plastics to make them more flexible, so present in many *plastic* products such as wall coverings, tablecloths, floor tiles, furniture upholstery, shower curtains, garden hoses, swimming pool liners, rainwear, baby pants, dolls, some toys, shoes, car/automobile upholstery, packaging film and sheets, sheathing for wires and cables, medical tubing, and blood storage bags.

Diethylene Glycol

Also known as 2,2'-dihydroxydiethyl ether. Used as a moistening agent for *tobacco*, *adhesives* and *paper* to stop them drying out. Also used as a softening agent for fabrics, and as a *solvent* for some dyes. Derivatives are used in *lacquers*.

Di-Glycerides Of Fatty Acids

See *mono and di-glycerides of fatty acids*.

Dihydroxyacetone

Also known as DHA. Used in sunless tanning lotions.

Dimethicone

A silicone oil. Typical products include hand cream, body lotion, shampoo, conditioner, moisturiser, after-shave, eye shadow and antacids. Also used as a barrier cream for industrial workers.

Dimethyl Dicarbonate
Used as a *yeast* inhibitor in *wine* and juices.

Dioctyl Phthalate
One of the most commonly used *plasticisers*.

Diphenyl
Used to stop fungus growing during the shipping of apples and oranges.

DMDM Hydantoin
A preservative that works by releasing *formaldehyde* into the product. Found in skin, body and hair products, antiperspirants and *nail polishes*.

Dishwasher Powders And Liquids
Similar ingredients to those in *detergents*, but sodium aluminate, boric oxide or aluminum phosphate may be added to reduce the risk of damage to the glaze on crockery. *Sodium carbonate, sodium hydroxide* or trisodium phosphate may be added to help remove grease. Traces will often remain on *crockery* and *cutlery*. This will be encountered outside the home in restaurants, etc., even if not used domestically.

Disodium Diphosphate
Also known as E450(i). A raising agent, *stabiliser* and emulsifier. Found in a wide range of foods including pastries, biscuits/cookies, desserts, protein drinks, etc.

Disodium EDTA
A *stabiliser* found in body washes, *hair dyes*, body lotions, shampoos and *cosmetics*.

Dog

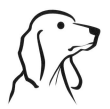

Major allergens in saliva, epidermal scales (*dander*) and urine. Less likely to be a problem than *cats* as they groom themselves less, and so spread less of the common protein allergens on to their fur.

Dralon

See *acrylic*.

Dried Fruit

Dried fruit is often sulphured (using *sulphur dioxide*) to keep it from oxidising during the drying process. Unsulphured fruit is generally browner and retains less of its original colour. Small quantities of *mineral oil* are often used to give sheen to the dried fruit. *Ethyl methanoate* may be used as a *fumigant*.

Drinking Water

See *water*.

Drugs

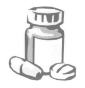

Can cause an allergic reaction either because of the drug itself or because of the ingredients that go to make up the tablets, liquid or cream. Many side effects of medicines are allergic reactions: if the allergy is removed, the side effects disappear too. When an individual has difficulty stopping a drug, this may be because they are allergic and addicted to it. Removing the allergy can simplify the process of stopping the drug. See also *tablets* and *capsules*.

Dry Cleaning

The main chemical used is *perchloroethylene*, but other chemicals (e.g. *trichloroethane*, ethylene dichloride, *naphtha*, *benzene*, and *toluene*) may also be used particularly for spot cleaning.

Dust

Dust can contain many things and the composition will be determined by many factors, e.g. whether the dust is outside or inside a building, what happens in the area, etc. See *house dust* and *particulate matter*.

Dyes

See *colouring*.

E

Edible Starch

See *modified starch*.

EDTA

See *disodium EDTA*.

Egg

In general egg whites are more likely to provoke problems than egg yolks. Egg white contains the proteins ovalbumin, ovomucoid and ovotransferrin, which seem to cause the most problems. Cooking changes ovalbumin and ovotransferrin, so that people sensitive to these proteins often do not react to well-cooked eggs. Some people allergic to chicken eggs are also allergic to *chicken*. The yolk may also contain *lutein* or *capsanthin*, as these are added to chicken feed to increase the colour of the egg yolk. Egg albumen is sometimes used in *wine* making to clear the wine.

Egg Beaters
A proprietary product made from *egg* white with added nutrients, including *beta carotene*.

Elastane
Also known as lycra and spandex. A man-made fibre based on *polyurethane*. Used to make bras, foundation garments, hosiery, tights/panty hose, sports clothes (including swim wear, ski pants, golf jackets, cycling clothes, and running shorts), and disposable nappies (diapers). Also found in *elastic* and sewing thread in other clothing and furnishings.

Elastic
Elastic used in clothes may contain *elastane, latex, lycra, thiuram* and *paraphenylenediamine*.

E Numbers
Method of labelling food additives used in the European Community. Also used in some other countries but without the E prefix, so E102 will be simply listed as 102, and so on. See also *FD & C numbers* and appendix 1.

Envelopes

The *glue* is usually made from *gum Arabic, gum tragacanth* or *tapioca* starch.

Emulsifiers

These are added to manufactured food (particularly low-calorie and low fat products), and personal care products to prevent water and oil separating. Also used in some industrial processes.

Epicoccum

A *mould* found on plants, in soil, grain, textiles and *paper* products. A common allergen.

Epoxy Resin

Used in *adhesives, paints* and in protective coatings, including those on metal cans.

Erythrosine

A cherry-red *food colouring* also known as E127, FD & C Red 3, Food Red 14 and C.I. 45430. Used in glacé cherries, confectionery, *baked goods*, snack foods, custard mix, processed meat products and *drugs*. Also used to reveal plaque in *dental* disclosing tablets. Banned in Norway, USA, Australia and New Zealand.

Ethanol

See *alcohol*.

Ethanolamine

Used in *detergents*, bactericidal and herbicidal products and *emulsifiers*. Also in the preparation of *cosmetics*, personal care products and *hair dyes*.

Ethene

See *ethylene*.

Ethenylbenzene

See *styrene*.

Ethoxydiglycol
Used as a *solvent* in hair lighteners, hair conditioners, *cosmetics* and personal care products.

Ethyl Acetate
Found in *perfumes*, perfumed products, *nail polishes*, and *nail polish removers*. Also used industrially as a *solvent* for *varnishes*, lacquers and nitrocellulose, and in the manufacture of *rayon* and *leather* and photographic films. Used in *decaffeination* of *tea* and *coffee*. In Australia, allowed as a carrier for food *flavourings*.

Ethyl Alcohol
See *alcohol*.

Ethylene
Given off in minute amounts by ripe tomatoes, bananas and *apples*. Also used commercially to encourage ripening in green bananas after shipping. Used extensively in the manufacturing of other chemicals (e.g. *ethanol*, *styrene*, etc.).

Ethylenediamine Dihydrochloride
An industrial *solvent*. Also found in eye drops, and as a preservative in some prescription skin creams.

Ethylene Dichloride
Also known as 1,2-dichloroethane. Used in the manufacture of *vinyl chloride*. Also an additive in *petrol* and so found in *vehicle exhaust fumes*.

Ethylene Glycol
Main ingredient in anti-freeze. Also used as a corrosion inhibitor to protect metal surfaces within cooling systems, and in the production of *polyester* and some *plasticisers*.

Ethylene Tetrachloride
See *perchloroethylene*.

Ethyl Formate
See *ethyl methanoate*.

Ethyl Methanoate
Also known as ethyl formate. Used as a *fumigant* for *tobacco, dried fruit* and other foodstuffs.

Ethyl Paraben
See *parabens*.

Ethyl Succinate
Also known as diethyl succinate. Used as a *fixative* for *perfumes*.

Eugenol
From clove oil. Used in dentistry, and also as *flavouring* and *perfume* in personal care products and food.

Expanded Plastics
Used in packaging. Made from *polystyrene, polyurethane, PVC, polyethylene, urea* and phenolic resins.

Fabrics
Fabrics can be made from a wide variety of materials. Problems can occur not only because of the material itself, but also because of *dyes* and finishes. If the fabric is minimum iron or flame-retardant, chemicals such as *formaldehyde* will be present. Dyes, c*hlorine* and optical brighteners will also be used to give the fabric a more

pleasing appearance. Chemicals such as *sodium hexametaphosphate* and *tannin* may also be used to fix the dyes. The thread used to sew fabric may not be of the same material as the fabric itself. The label on the fabric can still say '100% cotton' even if *polyester* threads, and

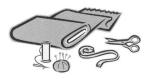

chemicals to achieve a particular look or finish have been used. See also *denim*.

Fake Tan Preparations

See *sun tan preparations*.

FD & C Colours

A classification used by the American Food & Drink Administration to categorise *colourings* that have been approved for use in foods, drugs and *cosmetics*. See also *D & C*. For individual colourings see appendix 1.

FD & C Green 3

A sea green *food colouring* also known as food green 3, C.I. 42053, and fast green FCF. This colouring does not have an *E number*. Found in beverages, desserts, confectionery and *baked goods*.

Feathers

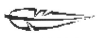

A common allergen that may be encountered in *bedding*, upholstery and some cold-weather clothing. People who keep birds as pets, or work with birds may also be affected.

Fish Paste

The names often suggests that these only contain one particular fish, but this may not be true, e.g. crab paste may contain mackerel and cod. The exact combination of fish is listed in the ingredients.

Fixative
A substance that holds another substance in position. Added to *perfumes* to delay evaporation of the perfume oils themselves, and to *fabric* dyes to increase colour-fastness.

Flavor
See *flavouring*.

Flavour
See *flavouring*.

Flavoured
See *flavouring*.

Flavour Enhancers
Added to food products to enhance the taste and palatability of a food without adding flavour in themselves. *Monosodium glutamate* is probably the best known.

Flavouring
These can be natural or synthetic. Many chemical substances used as both *flavourings* and *perfumes*. No standard list of food flavourings. Manufacturers have flavourings made up for specific products. Several products from the same manufacturer may be mint flavoured, but this does not mean that the mint flavouring used is identical in all the products. Product ingredient lists usually just say flavouring or natural flavouring or artificial flavouring. When the label says 'xx flavour' (e.g. strawberry flavour drink) product does not need to contain any xx, just taste as though it does. If says 'xx flavoured' (e.g. strawberry flavoured drink), a significant part of the flavour must come from xx. Manufacturers may vary the exact combination and quantity of flavourings they use to even-out normal variations in the flavour of natural ingredients.

Flour

Most flour is from *wheat*. Self-raising flour is made by adding *baking powder* to normal flour. See also *baked goods*.

Flourine

Used in some *plastics*, refrigerants, *aerosol propellants* and *toothpastes*. Also used in some areas for treating drinking *water*.

Flower Pollen

People often assume that an allergic reaction to flowers is to roses and similar plants with large flowers. This is unusual except in keen gardeners and florists. The flowers are large in order to attract pollinating insects that then carry the sticky pollen to another flower. This means that very little of the pollen is in the air, unlike smaller flowers which tend to be pollinated by the wind. Pollen from these often nondescript plants can travel long distances on the air currents and are most likely to be a problem. See also *pollens* and *tree pollens*.

Food Additive

Chemicals added to food to enhance colour, flavour, keeping qualities, etc.

Food Colouring

Many artificial food colourings are derived from *crude oil* and are known as *azo dyes*. Natural colours are often thought to be safe, but many people still react to them. This may be caused by the extraction process, as chemical *solvents* are used in this process. Non-food products may also contain artificial and natural food colourings, e.g. *cosmetics*, skin care products, *nutritional supplements* and *drugs*. In most countries food colourings are governed by legislation. There is no complete international agreement about which food colourings are safe; the list of accepted food colourings varies from country to country. Also see appendix 1.

Food Families

Foods are commonly divided up into food families: foods that are biologically alike. Many people are allergic to all or several members of the same food family, although it is possible to be allergic to only one member of the family. Some of the food families are well known, such as the grains (wheat, rice, barley etc.), but others like the deadly nightshade family, which includes potatoes, *tobacco*, tomatoes, red peppers etc. in its members, seem an odd assortment to those of us without the necessary botanical knowledge. The food families are listed in Appendix 2.

Food Flavourings

See *flavourings*.

Food Starch

See *starch*.

Footwear

Can involve *leather*, polyvinyl chloride, rubber, formaldehyde, *dyes*, etc.

Formaldehyde

Also known as methanal. One of the most common chemicals in the modern environment and a very common allergen. Can be released into the air by burning wood, kerosene or natural gas, in *vehicle exhaust fumes*, and by *tobacco smoke*. Used as a disinfectant, germicide, *fungicide*, defoamer and preservative (particularly for *cosmetics*, personal care products and *vaccines*). Also used as an industrial *adhesive* and so find its way into modern furniture, chipboard etc. Present in synthetic *rubber*, photographic chemicals, *paints*, upholstery, *washing up liquids*, slow-release fertilisers, *rayon* and *cavity wall insulation*. Increases the wet-strength of paper products, such as tissues and toilet rolls. Gives *fabrics* specialist finishes (e.g. minimum iron etc). Used in the

treatment of warts and verrucas. Used to preserve specimens for
biology classes and similar.

Formalin
A mixture of *formaldehyde* and *methanol*. The most common form
of formaldehyde in commercial use.

Fragrance
In the USA perfumes added to a product are called 'fragrance' on
the list of ingredients. In the European Community the word is
parfum. See *parfum* and *perfume*.

Fructose
Also known as fruit sugar. Found naturally in fruits, vegetables and
honey. Used commercially in *soft drinks* and diabetic foods.

Fruit Juices
 Fruit juices are often made from reconstituted juice. This
means that some of the water has been removed, the
remaining juice has been transported elsewhere and
water has been re-added. *Solvents* may also be used in
the extraction process and *silicone* anti-foam may be
added to control unwanted foam during the production process.
Some fruit drinks will have added *sugar*, *colourings* and
flavourings.

Fumigant
A chemical that is used in its gaseous state as a *fungicide*, e.g.
methyl bromide and *ethyl methanoate*.

Fungicides
Chemicals that inhibit fungal attack. Used food, including during
transportation and storage, and on wood and plastics, etc. Likely to
contain chemicals to aid spraying, as well as active ingredients.

Furniture Polish
May contain *ammonia, naptha, nitrobenzene*, petroleum distillates, *phenol*, and *perfume*, as well as various *waxes*.

G

Gammon
Gammon is the hind leg cut from a side of bacon after being mildly cured. See also *bacon* and *pork*.

Garlic
A member of the onion family, widely used in processed and restaurant food.

Gasoline
See *petrol*.

Gelatin / Gelatine
Comes from the bones, hooves, skin, tendons and ligaments of animals. People allergic to a particular meat are usually also allergic to gelatine derived from that animal. Used to thicken desserts such as jellies, yoghurt and confectionery. May be used in *wine* fining. The *capsules* used for *drugs* and *nutritional supplements* are usually made from gelatine. Also used in photography and the manufacture of some *adhesives*.

Genetically Modified Food
Genetically modified food contains genes derived from animals, fish, insects and bacteria. Genetic modifications are designed to transfer desirable qualities from one organism to another. There is concern that a person who is allergic to one thing would experience an allergic reaction on contact with a second substance containing a

genetic modification from the first. Governments tend to assume there is no difference between genetically engineered food and existing foods, so that it is not necessary to label a food or ingredient as genetically modified. In the UK, at least, the fact that a substance is not genetically modified is a selling point so this is being increasingly seen on food labels.

Geraniol

A synthetic chemical used as a general purpose *perfume* (rose and geranium) and *flavouring* (apple, blueberry, cherry, grapefruit, lemon, lime, orange, peach, pineapple, watermelon) in food, personal care products, *cosmetics* and household products.

Ghee

Clarified *butter* or, sometimes clarified *palm oil*, used in Indian cookery.

Gin

Distilled from malted *grain* and flavoured with juniper berries.

Glucose

Found naturally in honey and many fruits. Derived commercially from *corn,* (or occasionally from *wheat*). Used as a sweetener, so is found in confectionery, desserts, *ice cream*, *soft drinks* and drugs. Also produced in the body when complex sugars are converted into simpler sugars.

Glue

See *adhesives*.

Glutaraldehyde

Glutaraldehyde-based disinfectants used for cleaning and sterilising equipment and surfaces in hospitals, dentists, etc. Used in manufacture of *paper packaging* that will be in contact with food.

Gluten

Present in *wheat, barley* and *rye*; gives them their sticky quality when they are mixed with water. The harder varieties of wheat have more gluten. Durum wheat used to make pasta has the highest levels of gluten. Wheat used to make biscuits/cookies, cakes and pastries has the lowest levels of gluten. Lower levels of gluten in barley and rye. Some people are undoubtedly sensitive to gluten, but many people with grain sensitivity are reacting to some other constituent of the grain. Cereal binder, cereal filler, starch, cereal protein, *modified starch, edible starch, food starch*, rusk and vegetable protein may contain gluten. Some people also avoid *oats*, but a five-year study of coeliacs in Finland (M Uusitupa , et al. 'Gut' 2002; Volume 50) found that those who avoided oats experienced no significant difference in their intestinal health compared to those who did not.

Glycerin

See *glycerol*.

Glycerol

Also known as glycerine and E422. Can be produced artificially from propylene alcohol, or naturally derived from *vegetable oils* or animal sources. Used in the manufacture of inks, lubricants, explosives, personal care products (e.g. *toothpastes*, moisturisers, shower gels, hair products), and *cosmetics*. Also used as a sweetening agent in *drugs* (e.g. ear drops and cough mixtures). In food it is found in confectionery, cereal bars, desserts, soft-scoop *ice cream* and many alcoholic drinks. Also used in *gelatine capsules*, and as a moistening agent for *tobacco* (to keep it from drying out).

Glycerol Monostearate

Used widely in food production, e.g. to keep *baked goods* fresh, as a flour improver, in *ice cream, chewing gum*, desserts, *chocolates* and *cosmetics*.

Glyceryl Stearate
Found in personal care products, such as cleansers, face wash creams, body lotions, *sunscreens*, foundation and hair conditioners.

Glycol Distearate
Widely used to make *cosmetics* opaque.

Glycolic Acid
Used in *cosmetics* and personal care preparations, particularly skin peel preparations.

Goat's Milk
The two main proteins in milk are *casein* and *whey*. Casein in goat's and *cow's milk* are similar, but the whey differs. Individuals sensitive to the whey in cow's milk may be able to tolerate goat's milk.

Gold
A precious metal found in *dental* work and jewellery. Gold salts are used for treating rheumatoid arthritis. Can be used as a *food colouring*, but for external decoration only.

Grains
 Seeds of members of the grass family (see appendix 2). Some of these contain *gluten*.

Gram Flour
Made from chickpeas and used in Indian cookery.

Grass
Many people react to grass. In the UK the most common grasses that cause problems are perennial rye grass (Lolium perenne) and

timothy grass (Phleum pratense). Many people react adversely when grass is cut. They often assume this is because they are allergic to grass pollens, but it could equally well be *moulds*. Moulds grow in the matted layer at the base of the grass blades and are disturbed and released into the atmosphere when the grass is cut. In the UK grass pollen is common from May to August with a peak in June and early July. Some people who are allergic to grass pollen will also react to *wheat*, *rye* and *corn* when eaten. See appendix 3 for a pollen calendar.

Green S

A *food colouring* also known as E142, Acid Brilliant Green BS, Lissamine Green , Food Green 4 and C.I. 44090. Used in confectionery, desserts, *ice cream*, tinned peas, packet bread crumbs, mint sauce and gravy granules. Banned in Canada, Finland, Japan, Norway, Sweden and the United States.

Green Peppers

 Unripe version of red, yellow and orange peppers.

Groundnut Oil

Made from *peanuts*.

Guar Gum

Also known as E412. A *stabiliser* extracted from the seed of the leguminous shrub Cyamopsis tetragonoloba. Commonly found in salad dressings, dips, mayonnaise, milk shakes, *ice cream* and desserts. Also used in *paper* manufacturing, textiles, printing, *cosmetics* and *drugs*.

Gum Acacia

See *gum Arabic*.

Gum Arabic

Also known as E414 and gum acacia. A *stabiliser* made from the acacia tree. Used in *soft drinks* and *beers* (to stabilise the foam), in glazes and toppings for *baked goods* where it acts as an adhesive, in meal replacement drinks, and as an emulsifying and suspending agent in *drugs*. Also used for the glue on *stamps*, and in *water colour paints*.

Gum Karaya

Also known as sterculia gum. A natural product from the sterculia tree. Used to prevent large crystals forming in water ices, etc. Also used to bind water in meat products and cheese spreads, and as a dental adhesive and a laxative.

Gum Tragacanth

Also known as E413. Plant derived. Widely used including for salad dressings, *ice cream*, *drugs*, *cosmetics*, and the glue on *stamps* and *envelopes*.

Gypsum

Also known as selenite. Used in the production of plaster and plasterboard – most internal walls are lined with plasterboard. Also use in plaster of Paris, and to control the setting rate of Portland *cement*, and as a filler.

H

Ham
Traditionally ham is produced by trimming *pork*, salting the skin and exposed meat heavily and hanging it in an airy space so that the salt draws the moisture out and the flesh absorbs the salt back in. In mass-produced ham *sodium nitrate* and *sodium nitrite* often used.

Hair Colouring
See *hair dyes*.

Hair Dyes
These may contain a whole range of different chemicals. Common ones include *hydrogen peroxide*, *ammonia* and *para-phenylenediamine*.

Halazone
Used in the sterilisation of drinking *water*.

Haloacetic Acids
Produced as a by-product of *water* sterilisation.

Heating Fumes
Fumes from burning gas, oil, coal and wood in heating systems. Can be highly allergenic for some people.

Heptane
A *solvent* used in the production of oils, and in manufacture of *adhesives*.

Herbal Supplements
Those supplied for the mass market may use chemical *solvents* to extract the maximum amount of the active ingredient from the herb.

As this is part of the production process, they do not need to be included in the list of ingredients. See also *herbs*, *tablets* and *capsules*.

Herbal Teas

Many people think these are non-allergenic but it is possible to be allergic to the *herbs*, *flavourings*, or the *paper* and *adhesive* of the tea bag.

Herbs

Herbs are in a variety of botanical families, so it is rare for someone to react to all herbs, but it is common for people to react to individual herbs. I was allergic to chamomile, but did not know this. I bought some washing up liquid containing chamomile. In the following week I felt sick every time I ate, the roof of my mouth became covered with blisters, my joints started to ache and I felt extremely tired. I thought I was seriously ill until I found that I was highly allergic to chamomile and minute traces on cutlery and crockery were enough to give me these alarming symptoms.

Hexane

A widely used industrial chemical used, for example, in *pesticide* manufacture, as a cleaning agent in the printing industry, and as a *solvent* for *varnishes* and *adhesives*.

High Density Polyethylene

Also known as HDPE. See *polyethylene*.

Histamine

Some foods such as *wine* and *cheese* naturally contain high levels of histamine. See also pages 5 and 18.

Homosalate
See *trimethylsiloxysilicate*.

Honey
Varies tremendously depending on the source of the nectar for the

bees. Many types of honey will contain minute
quantities of *flower pollens*. People with hay fever
may react to these pollens. Yet many hay fever
sufferers find taking small quantities of local honey
throughout the hay fever season helps to control
their hay fever. The pollens in the honey seem to be
acting like a homeopathic desensitising programme.

Hops
In the same botanical family as figs and mulberry. Used in *beer*.

Hot Tubs
See *swimming pool water*.

House Dust
A mixture of many substances. May contain *moulds*, fabric fibres,
human hair, skin particles, *house dust mites*, food particles and other
debris, and *dander* from *dogs*, *cats*, and other animals. Will also
contain particles brought into home on shoes and clothes, and
pollution, *pollens*, etc. blown in from outside. Content varies from
home to home, depending on type of furniture, building materials,
insulation, presence of *pets*, the neighbourhood, the weather and
other factors. A person may be allergic to one or more of these
substances. As well as being a problem for some people in its own
right, dust particles act as carriers for other substances, such as *lead*,
allowing them to enter the respiratory system. See also *particulate
matter*.

House Dust Mite

Related to spiders and ticks, but so small that they cannot be seen by the naked eye. Found in every home, particularly in *mattresses* and *bedding*. Millions of mites in a bed. The number of mites in the average house appears to be increasing as central heating and fitted carpets provide an ideal environment for them. The mite feeds on the dead skin that we shed constantly. Often the allergy is not to the house dust mite itself but to its faecal droppings. Many people with *eczema* are sensitive to the house dust mite or its droppings. As they lie in bed scratching, they produce an abundant supply of food for the mite, but even people without eczema shed minute flakes of skin constantly. As well as being a trigger for eczema, the house dust mite will often affect *asthma* and *allergic rhinitis* sufferers. People who wake with a blocked nose or start the day with a *sneezing* fit often are reacting to it. An allergy to the mite will cause some people to snore. People who are allergic to house dust mite and *shrimp* and *prawns* are reacting to a muscle protein they all share. If the person is sensitive to some other part of the house dust mite, they will not necessarily also react to shrimp and prawn. Washing sheets and bedding at over 60°C will kill house dust mites. Also see *storage mite*.

Hydrazine

Used in various industrial processes, including nickel-plating.

Hydrocarbons

Chemical compounds that contain hydrogen and carbon. *Petrol* and *diesel* are hydrocarbon fuels, as are many of the basic chemicals used by industry to make *plastics*, *waxes* and oils.

Hydrogenated Vegetable Oils

Vegetable oils are generally liquid at room temperature. Food manufacturers often want a solid fat that does not go rancid easily, so liquid vegetable oils are heated to high temperatures and a catalyst (commonly *nickel*, but could be *palladium*, *platinum* or rhodium) is added. Hydrogen is bubbled through the liquid. The mixture is then filtered to remove the metal, leaving hydrogenated vegetable oil, which is solid at room temperature and has a long shelf life.

Hydrogen Peroxide
Used in chemical production and *pollution* control. Found in cleaning products as a disinfectant and deodoriser. Also used in food bleaching, *hair dyes*, and the textile and *paper* industries. In the body involved in destruction of pathogens by white blood cells.

Hydrogen Sulphide
Very toxic gas that smells like rotten eggs in low concentrations. Produced during the decomposition of organic matter such as sewage and animal manure, in vehicle exhaust fumes and occasionally in home wine making.

Hydrolised Collagen
Collagen that has been broken down partly or completely into its constituent amino acids. In skin creams, nail care products and hair treatments.

Hydroxycitronellal
Widely used to impart a floral *perfume* in personal care products and *cosmetics*. Also used as a *flavouring* in food. May be found in some antiseptics and *insecticides*.

Hydroxyethylcellulose
Found in personal care products (e.g. hair conditioners, body toning creams, *mascaras* and shaving creams). Also used in dry-eye medication.

Hydroxymethylglycinate
Found in personal care products (e.g. cleansing lotions, toning lotions, eye gels, moisturisers, shampoos and pre-shave lotions).

Hydroxypropyl Methylcellulose
From *cellulose*. Used to make *capsules*.

I

Ice Cream
May contain a variety of ingredients including *cow's milk*, cream, *sugar, glucose, flavourings, colourings, emulsifiers* (e.g. *polysorbate 80*), *stabilisers* (e.g. *sodium alginate*), etc.

Imidazolidinyl Urea
A preservative found in skin, body and hair products, antiperspirants and *nail polishes*.

Indigo
Originally plant based, but now produced almost entirely synthetically using *naphthalene, cinnamic acid, sodium hydroxide* and other chemicals. Used to dye cotton cloth to create *denim*.

Indigo Carmine
A royal blue *food colouring* also known as E132, Indigotine, FD & C Blue No 2, Food Blue 1 and C.I. 73015. Commonly found in *baked goods*, cereals, snack foods, *ice cream* and confectionery. Often added to medicinal *tablets* and *capsules*. Used diagnostically in kidney function tests. Banned in Norway.

Indigotine
See *indigo carmine*.

Industrial Chemicals

 There are some chemicals that are widely used in industrial processes (e.g. *triethanolamine, dimethylamine, formaldehyde, phenol* and *ethanol*). Correcting one of these, may result in reactions to a wide range of products being corrected.

Insect Bite/Sting

Many insect stings or bites cause a 'normal' reaction, but in people who are allergic to them the incident produces a much stronger reaction usually involving itching and extensive swelling in the area. This may last for several days. In severe cases *anaphylactic shock* may result. See also *bee sting* and *wasp sting*.

Insecticide

Chemicals used to kill insects. See also *pesticides*.

Insect Repellants

May contain butopyronoxyl, cimethyl phthalate, diethyltoluamide (DEET), diethyl toluanide, dimethyl phthlate, ethyl hexanediol, indalone, di-n-propylisocinchoronate, bicycloheptene dicarboximide, and tetrahydro furaldehyde.

Inulin

A *starch* found in numerous edible plant species including chicory, artichoke, leek, onion, asparagus, *wheat, barley, rye, garlic,* and *bananas*. Used in processed foods including some *margarine*, yoghurt and confectionery.

Invertase

A yeast-derived enzyme that improves the shelf life of confectionery, particularly soft-centred chocolates.

Irish Moss
See *carageenan*.

Iron
A metal found in granite, sandstone and most *clays*. *Steel* is made from it. See also *iron oxide*.

Iron Oxide
Also known as rust. Used as a colour in *lipstick*, medicinal *tablets*, toner for *photocopiers* and printers, *paints* and *plastics*, ceramic magnets, and as a *tattoo* dye.

Isinglass
From the swim bladders of fish, used in *wine* fining.

Isobutane
An *aerosol propellant* commonly found in hair sprays etc. Also used as a refrigerant in freezers and fridges.

Isoeugenol
A commonly used *perfume* in personal care products. Also used in the manufacture of *vanillin*.

Isopropyl
See *alcohol*.

Isopropyl Acetate
Used as a *solvent* for *perfume*. Found in cleaning fluids, printing ink, *cosmetics* and personal care products.

Isopropyl Isostearate
Frequently used in skin care products and *cosmetics*.

Isopropyl Myristate
Found in hand and body lotions, moisturisers, deodorants, body sprays, pre-shave lotions, *mascara* and *perfumes*.

Isopropyl Palminate
Frequently found in *cosmetics* and personal care preparations.

Isothiazolinone
Preservative in oil and cooking fluids, *soaps*, *detergents*, shampoos, hair conditioners, bubble baths, skin creams and lotions, *mascaras*, baby wipes, etc.

J

Japan Wax
A wax obtained from the berries of a plant (sumac). Used in polishes and eyebrow pencils.

Jewellery

 Made from a variety of different materials including *gold*, *silver*, *nickel*, glass, *plastic*, precious and semi-precious stones, etc.

Joint Replacements
A combination of metal (*stainless steel*, alloys of *cobalt* and *chrome*, or *titanium*) and *polyethylene* is usually used. As the polyethylene wears, microscopic particles can become loose and damage the bone and surrounding tissue.

Jojoba Oil

An oil extracted from a shrub. Used in hair care products, *cosmetics* and skin care preparations.

Jute

A fibre made from a plant grown in Asia; used as a backing for *carpets*, and sacks for carrying grains, fertilisers and cement.

K

Kaolin

A type of fine *clay*. May be found in face masques, *toothpastes* and *anti-caking agents*. Used as a filler in *paper*. A relatively new use is as a pest control particularly for grapes, apples and citrus fruit.

Kapok

Made from the floss that covers the seed pods of the silk-cotton tree (ceiba tree). Found in cushions and soft toys, although use is declining, as being replaced by *polyester*.

Kerosene

Another name for *paraffin*.

Kipper

A smoked herring.

L

Lacquer
Natural or synthetic *resins* dissolved in a *solvent* that evaporates rapidly leaving a shiny coating.

Lactalbumin
One of the proteins in *milk*.

Lactic Acid
Also known as E270. Typical products include meat extracts, pickled onions, *margarine*, desserts, confectionery, sports drinks, and personal care products (e.g. cleansing lotion, toning lotion, eye gel, shampoo, pre-shave lotion). Also used in vaginal douches and wart treatments. Used industrially in *textile* finishing and in *leather* tanning. Also occurs naturally in muscles during periods of physical exertion.

Lactoglobulin
One of the principal proteins in *milk*.

Lactose
One of the sugars present in *milk*, which is broken down by the enzyme lactase. Lactose intolerance occurs where the body is not able to produce lactase. Without this, lactose ferments in the bowel causing various health problems. Estimated that about 4-6% of the Anglo white population are lactose intolerant. The numbers are much higher among Africans and Asians. Found in *cow's milk*, *goat's milk*, and *sheep's milk*. Fermented products (such as yoghurt) are usually tolerated well. Hard *cheese* contains very little lactose and so may be tolerated. Used as an ingredient in its own right in packet sauces, desserts, *chocolate*, antacid preparations and medicinal tablets.

Lager

A blonde *beer* fermented for a longer time and at a lower temperature than normal beer. The *yeast* used is Saccharomyces uvarum.

Lanolin

Also known as wool alcohol. Produced by the oil glands of sheep. Obtained commercially from sheep's *wool*, and is. A very common allergen. Found in *cosmetics*, personal care products (including *lip balms*), *soap* and wool. May also be found in printing inks and *paper*. May be used in medicinal ointments and creams, particularly those used to treat *eczema* and *dermatitis*.

Lanolin Alcohol

Derived from *lanolin*, but with fewer allergy problems. Used in *cosmetics*, skin care and depilatory creams.

Lard

Made from *pork* fat. May be used in pastry and for frying, although its use has declined dramatically in recent years.

Latex

A rubber derivative. Can be either natural or synthetic. Natural latex made from sap of rubber tree. Synthetic latex made from *neoprene*, *nitrile*, etc. Found in protective gloves, coatings for *paper*, contraceptives (*condoms*, diaphragms and caps), hot water bottles, baby bottle teats, *shoes*, *mattresses*, *pillows*, balloons, rubber bands, *elastic* and finger stalls. Has a similar enzyme to ones found in kiwi, chestnut, banana and avocado, so, if this is the problem with the latex, the person will also show an allergic reaction to these. The powder that is used to dust the inside of latex gloves and condoms and make them easier to put on can be the cause of the problem rather than the latex itself. This is often *cornstarch* or silica, possibly with a small amount of magnesium oxide. Has been shown that sometimes the powder from medical gloves circulates in the air conditioning system and causes problems for people in that environment who are not wearing the gloves. Latex proteins can be present as 'hidden ingredients' in food, because people involved in the food preparation wear latex gloves (Dr. Roberto Bernardini et al, 'Journal of Allergy and Clinical Immunology', September 2002. See also *rubber*.

Laundry Detergents
See *detergents*.

Lauramide DEA
Produced from *coconut* oil. Used in *soaps* and *cosmetics*. Under certain circumstances may produce *nitrosamines*.

Laureth-23
Used in skin care products.

L-Cysteine Hydrochloride
Also known as E920. Can be from vegetarian or non-vegetarian sources. Used as a flour treatment agent, so may be in *bread*, pastry, etc.

Lead
A heavy metal found in old water pipes, old paint, improperly glazed pottery, *cigarette* ash, old *pewter*, lead crystal ware and *pollution* from waste incinerators. Because of restrictions on using lead as a petrol/gas additive, levels of airborne lead have declined, but there are still deposits of lead in the ground near busy traffic areas, and at times this can become airborne. Not used in pewter now because of health concerns.

Lead Acetate
Used in *hair dyes*, particularly those for grey hair that take effect over a number of washes.

Leather
Usually pig or cow hide. Sodium sulphide and *calcium hydroxide* are usually used to remove hair. Treated with *chromates*, *tannin*, *acetaldehyde*, *dyes*, *waxes*, etc.

Lecithin
Also known as E322. Made from *eggs*, sunflower or most commonly *soya*. An antioxidant/ emulsifier commonly used in cakes, confectionery, gravy granules, *margarine*, cereal bars, and instant powdered products.

Lettuce
 Part of an extensive food family that includes sunflower, sesame, artichoke and *ragweed*. A surprisingly large number of people are allergic to lettuce.

Limonene
The major constituent of citrus essential oils, used as a raw material for the chemical synthesis of *terpene*, *adhesives* and *flavourings* (e.g. menthol), so a common ingredient in *perfumed* products.

Linalool
One of the most frequently used *perfumes*. May be from natural sources (e.g. basil or lavender) or synthetic. Found in personal care products, *cosmetics* and household products.

Linen
A fabric made from the flax plant. By-products of linen production are processed into a pulp used for *banknotes* and fibreboard.

Lip Balm
The use of lip balms has dramatically increased. It is interesting that many people with food allergies suffer with sore lips, and so feel a need to use these lip balms (see page 26). Sometimes they turn out also to be allergic to the lip balm. Common ingredients include *oxybenzone, octyl methoxycinnamate, mineral oil* and *lanolin*.

Lipstick

Because lipstick is on the lips a large quantity of it ends up in the digestive system. Ingredients include oils and waxes (particularly castor oil, but also olive oil, sunflower oil, cocoa butter, *lanolin, mineral oil, beeswax, candelilla wax, carnauba wax*, etc.), moisturisers, *sunscreens, colours* (e.g. *titanium dioxide, iron oxide, tartrazine*, etc.), preservatives (e.g. *BHA* and *propyl paraben*) and *flavourings*. Long-lasting colour lipsticks contain *silicone* oil, which seals the colour to the lips. Lip-gloss usually has less wax and more oils.

Liquid Soap

A *detergent* rather than a true *soap*. Likely to contain *sodium laureth sulphate, sodium lauryl sulphate* and *cocamidopropyl betaine*.

Locust Bean Gum
Also known as E410, carob bean gum and carubin. Used in dips, sausages, cream cheese, frozen desserts and *ice creams*.

Low Density Polyethylene
Also known as LDPE. See *polyethylene*.

Lutein
Also known as E161b. A *food colouring* that may
be used in chicken feed to give a dark yolk to the
eggs. Also used in desserts.

Lye
Also known as *sodium hydroxide* and *potassium hydroxide*.

Lycra
DuPont's brand name for *elastane*.

M

Mace
The outer casing of a nutmeg. Used in savoury dishes.

Magnesium Phosphates
See *anti-caking agents*.

Magnesium Stearate
Used as a gelling agent to produce industrial greases. Also found in
paints, *varnishes*, *lacquers*, *rubber*, candles, face and body powders,
and medicinal *tablets*.

Magnesium Stearate Hydroxide
See *talc*.

Maize
See *corn*.

Make-Up

See *cosmetics*.

Malt

Derived from sprouted and kiln-dried *barley*. Used as a *flavouring* in some beers, *bread* and breakfast cereals. Also may be found in vegetable mince (*meat substitute*).

Maltodextrin

Easily digestible carbohydrate made from natural *corn* starch (or occasionally from *wheat*). Not produced from and does not contain *malt* in spite of its name. Typical products include, infant foods, bakery goods, desserts, sports drinks and *drugs*.

Manganese

Used as a *colouring* and a bleaching agent. Also used in the manufacture of batteries, *steel* and *aluminium*. An alloy of manganese and *bronze* is used for some *coins*.

Mannitol

Also known as E421. Used medicinally as a diuretic, as a dietetic sweetener, and as the coating dust on *chewing gum*. Manufactured commercially by processing *glucose*, *fructose* and *sucrose*. Occurs naturally in the wood of coniferous trees.

Margarine

Made from *vegetable oils* that have been neutralised, bleached and deodorised to remove all colour, taste, smells and impurities. The oil is *hydrogenated* to make it the right texture. Water, *whey*, salt, vitamins, *colourings*, *flavourings* and *emulsifiers* are then added. Margarine products that have less than 80 percent oil are commonly called 'spreads' or low-fat, or reduced-fat margarine.

Mascara

May contain *beeswax*, *carnauba wax*, *stearic acid*, *parabens*, *titanium dioxide*, *iron oxide*, chromium hydroxide, *isopropyl myristate*, *triethanolamine*, vitamins, etc. *Nylon* used for lengthening fibres.

Mattresses

May include latex (synthetic or natural), *steel* springs, *polyurethane* foam, *nylon*, cotton, wool, plastic, etc. See also *beds and bedding*.

MEA

See *monoethanolamine*.

Meat

Different meats are in different food families (see appendix 2), so it is unusual to be allergic to all meat.

Meat Substitutes

Main ingredients are commonly *soya*, *wheat*, *yeast extract*, *flavourings* and herbs and spices.

Medication

See *drugs*.

Medicinal Tablets

See *tablets*.

Mercaptobenzothiazole

Found in flea sprays and powders, *rubber* products and *adhesives*.

Mercury

A toxic metal found in *dental amalgam*, *pesticides*, *fungicides*, *vaccines*, emissions from coal-burning power stations and contaminated fish. See also *dental amalgam*.

Methanol

Also known as methyl alcohol, wood alcohol, wood spirits, or curbinol. Used in the industrial production of many synthetic organic compounds and constituent of many *solvents*. Used to make *formaldehyde*. Typical products include windscreen/windshield wiper fluids and de-icers, antifreeze, glass cleaners, *paints*, *varnishes*, paint thinners and removers.

Methylene Chloride

Also known as methylene dichloride and dichloromethane. Commonly found in septic tank cleaners, *paint* and *varnish* removers, *degreasers*, *pesticides*, *aerosols*, and Christmas bubble lights. Also used as a *solvent* in coffee and tea *decaffeination*, and in *perfumed* products.

Methyl Alcohol

See *methanol*.

Methyl Paraben

See *parabens*.

Methyl Salicylate

The principal constituent of oil of wintergreen and oil of sweet birch. Found in artificial *flavours*, sports rubs and pain relief creams. Also used as a *perfume*.

Methyl Trichloride

See *trihalomethanes*.

Mica

A mineral used to give a pearly effect to *cosmetics* and *nail polishes*.

Microcrystalline Wax

Derived from *petroleum*, used in skin care, *cosmetics* and *nail polishes*.

Microcrystalline Cellulose

Produced from high-quality wood pulp. Usually involves a strong acid such as hydrogen chloride. May be found in medicinal *tablets*, reduced-fat salad dressings, frozen desserts, whipped toppings, and bakery products.

Microfibre

Extremely fine extruded filaments of *polyester*, *nylon*, *acrylic*, or *rayon* fibres, which are made into *fabrics* mainly for clothing.

Mildew

This term is often used interchangeably with *mould*.

Milk

See *cow's milk*, *goat's milk*, *sheep's milk*, *casein*, *whey* and *lactose*.

Millet

A *grain* that is *gluten*-free.

Mineral Oil

Also known as paraffin oil; liquid petrolatum, white mineral oil and nujol. A derivative of *crude oil*. Used in wash water for sliced potatoes, on fruits and vegetables, coating on *dried fruit*, in the manufacture of *vinegar* and *wine*, in/on *capsules* and *tablets*, as a releasing agent in commercial baking trays, and in confectionery. Also used as a dust control agent for wheat, corn, soybean, barley, rice, rye, oats, & sorghum. Used generally as lubricant on food-processing equipment.

Mineral Oil Jelly
See *paraffinum liquidum*.

Modified Starch
A cheap filler, used to bulk out products. Produced by treating starch from various sources with acids, alkalis and oxidising agents to make it more soluble, or heat resistant, or to give it a variety of textures. Also used as an adhesive in cardboard manufacture. See also *starch*.

Mohair
Wool from the angora goat.

Molasses
Also known as treacle. Produced by boiling down juices from *sugar*, usually sugar cane, but could be sugar beet or maple.

Mold
See *moulds (airborne)* and *moulds(food)*.

Molybdenum
A metal used in *stainless steel*. Also used in *paints* and inks, *plastic* and *rubber* products, and ceramics. An additive in lubricants, including vehicle engine oil (as a sulphide). Also sold as *a nutritional supplement*.

Mono & Di-Glycerides Of Fatty Acids
Also known as E471. *Emulsifiers* in *margarine*, desserts, and ready meals.

Monoethanolamine
Also known as MEA. Found in personal care products. Under certain circumstances may produce *nitrosamines*.

Monosodium Glutamate

Also known as E621 and MSG. A *flavour enhancer* commonly found in processed meat products, gravy powder, stock cubes, tinned soup, crisps, fast food and some *Chinese food*. Originally made from seaweed, now made by a fermenting process using *starch*, *sugar* beets, sugar cane, or *molasses*.

Mortar

Made from *cement* and sand and used in stonework and brickwork.

Moulds (Airborne)

Related to yeasts and fungi. Can be a problem both indoors and outdoors. Will flourish in warm, moist conditions, and are a particular problem in basements, bathrooms, kitchens, greenhouses, *swimming pools*, saunas, and similar environments. Also a problem in *air conditioning* systems. Houseplants tend to increase the problem of moulds. One less commonly recognised source of mould spores is in lawns. As the *grass* is cut, mould spores will be released into the air from the damp, protected surface layer of soil. Outdoors, wet weather favours mould growth, and sunny windy weather favours the release of mould spores. The common airborne moulds in the U.K. include *alternaria*, *aspergillus*, *cladosporium*, *mucor* and *penicillium*. Other moulds found where water has been standing a long time include fusarium, trichoderma, and *stachybotrys*. Particularly implicated in *allergic rhinitis*, *asthma*, and respiratory problems generally. Because mould spores are small, it is possible for them to reach the finer tubes in the lungs.

Moulds (Food)

Present on foods long before they are visible to the naked eye, so a reaction to a food may be a reaction to a mould on the food rather than the food itself. Foods which are a particular problem include fruits (particularly soft fruit), *cheese*, nuts and seeds.

Mosquito

 A severe reaction to mosquito bites is usually a sign of an allergy to it. Anecdotal evidence that taking vitamin B complex minimises the number of bites people receive, although it does not reduce the severity of any reaction.

Mucor

A type of *mould* found in soil, horse dung, and on leather and decaying fruit and vegetables.

MSG

See *monosodium glutamate*.

Mugwort Pollen

Individuals who are sensitive to mugwort pollen may also react to celery, carrot, apple, spices, melon and chamomile as they share some of the same biochemical markers.

Municipal Water

See *water*.

Mushroom

A fungus, so related to *moulds*. People who are sensitive to moulds may also be sensitive to mushrooms.

Musk Ambrette

A synthetic chemical used in *perfumes*, incense sticks and personal care products.

Myristyl Myristate
Derived from *coconut* oil and used in *cosmetics* (particularly foundation and *lipsticks*), and skin care products.

N

Nail Polish

Common ingredients include toluenesulfonamide-*formaldehyde* resin, *xylene, acrylates copolymer*, acetyl tributyl citrate, *alcohol, butyl acetate, DMDM hydantoin, ethyl acetate* and *imidazolidinyl urea*. Colours (e.g. *titanium dioxide, D & C* Red 6) are also used. Bismuth oxychloride may be included to give a pearlised finish. Dibutyl phthalate (DBP), used to reduce chipping, was banned in Europe in 2004 because of health concerns, but still used elsewhere.

Nail Polish Remover
Likely to contain *acetone* or *ethyl acetate*.

Nail Varnish
See *nail polish*.

Naphthalene
Also known as tar camphor. Used as a pest repellent and is frequently found in mothballs, toilet bowl deodorisers, and carpet cleaners. Released when wood, *tobacco* and fossil fuels are burnt. Used to make many widely used chemicals, including synthetic *indigo*.

Naphthas

Derived from both *petroleum* distillation and *coal tar*. Used as organic *solvents* for dissolving or softening *waxes*, oils, greases, *varnishes*, and *plastics*. Also used in *dry cleaning* and *insecticides*.

Natural

In most countries this either has no legal standing, or else means much less than most consumers think. See also *natural food colourings* and *nature identical substances*.

Natural Food Colourings

Because of the concern about *food colourings*, many manufacturers are now using food colourings derived from natural sources, e.g. E162 made from beetroot, and E160(c) made from paprika. Common allergens, possibly because of the *solvents* used in extraction.

Nature Identical Substances

Although manufacturers claim that certain chemically produced substances are 'nature identical', this does not mean that the body reacts in exactly the same way to both.

Neoprene

Found in waterproof clothing and wet suits. Used to make synthetic *latex*.

Newsprint

Usually *carbon black* ink. Contains carbon black colour with a carrier (usually *petroleum* or *soya* based), anti-misting and low-rub 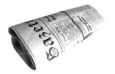 chemicals, and *paraffin* distillates for quick drying. Many coloured inks contain the same basic ingredients except pigments replace the carbon black to achieve the desired colour.

Nickel

A metal found in cheap jewellery, jean studs, hairpins, zips (zippers), bra clasps, buckles, keys, spectacles, *coins*, *stainless steel* and *hair dyes*. Also used as a catalyst for *hydrogenating vegetable oils*. The electrical

 elements in kettles and water heaters also contain nickel. Hot drinks made from water boiled in a kettle will contain minute traces of nickel. May be in flour as a result of milling. Nickel is present in the body in small amounts and is thought to activate certain enzymes. Nickel allergies are often aggravated by sweating.

Nicotine

Found in *tobacco* and some *pesticides*.

Nitrates

From nitrogenous fertilisers which are used in large quantities. May find their way into drinking *water*. Also found as *sodium nitrate* and *potassium nitrate* in food, etc.

Nitrile

A form of synthetic *rubber*. Oil and *solvent* resistant. Used to make washers, *rubber gloves*, and in *mattresses*, etc.

Nitrobenzene

Found in some *shoe polishes*, furniture polishes and floor polishes, leather dressings, *paints*, *solvents*, and sometimes used to mask unpleasant odours.

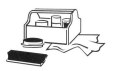

Nitrocellulose

Derived from *cellulose*. Used in *plastics*, *lacquers*, *nail polishes* and photographic film.

Nitrogen Dioxide
A major form of *air pollution*, mainly from traffic, power stations and other industrial sources.

Nitrogen Trichloride
When *chlorine* reacts with urine in *swimming pools* this chemical is produced.

Nitrosamines
Compounds formed when *nitrates* (usually from food or drinking water) react with *amines* naturally present in food and in the human body. Also found in some personal care products, and *tobacco smoke*. Between 1994 and 1997 a survey by UK government found more than half the *cosmetics* and personal care products surveyed contained detectable levels of nitrosamines. This included baby products. Not intentionally added to cosmetics, but are formed accidentally during manufacture or storage. Levels increase over time. Able to penetrate the skin.

Nutmeg
A spice used in cakes, biscuits and desserts.

Nutritional Supplements
As well as containing the actual vitamins and minerals, supplements contain diluents, coatings, *plasticisers*, disintegrants and lubricants. All of these can cause problems for sensitive people. See also *tablets* and *capsules*.

Nuts
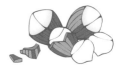
Different nuts are in different botanical families (see Appendix 2), but some people react to all or most nuts. This is likely to be because nuts have the same natural bacterial and fungicidal compounds that reduce rotting in damp soil, even though they are from different botanical families.

Nylon

Various types of nylon, e.g. nylon 6 and nylon 66. Very occasionally people allergic to only one type. Found in clothing, tights/panty hose and stockings, *carpets*, *mattresses* and furnishings, brushes, tyres, hoses, seat belts, parachutes, racket strings, ropes, nets, sleeping bags, tarpaulins, tents, thread, mono-filament fishing line, and dental floss. Used in some *mascaras* that contain thickening fibres.

O

Oak Moss

A 'masculine' *perfume* derived from lichen, used in men's personal care products and earthy, woody perfumes.

Oats

A *grain* used in porridge, muesli, granola and other cereals, biscuits, cereal bars and some specialist breads.

Ocimene

A widely used *perfume* in *cosmetics*, personal care products and household products.

Octyl Dodecanol

A common ingredient in *cosmetics*, hair conditioners and nail care products.

Octyl Gallate

Also known as E311. An *antioxidant* found in *margarine*, *peanut* butter, *cosmetics* (especially *lipsticks*) and medicinal creams.

Octyl Methoxycinnamate
Frequently found in *sunscreens* and *lip balms*.

Octyl Palmitate
Used in shaving creams, moisturisers and *lipsticks*.

Octyl Salicitate
An active ingredient in many *sunscreen preparations*.

Offices
The air in offices can contain many different chemicals, e.g. *ozone, triphenyl phosphate*, *perfumes* and *detergents* used by other people, *moulds* from the *air conditioning system* etc. New carpets and furniture will give off *volatile organic compounds*.

Oil Extraction (From Seeds)
See *vegetable oils*.

Olefin
See *polypropylene*.

Orange B
A *food colouring* used in the USA. The US FDA restricts its use to hot dogs and sausage casings.

Organic
In most countries personal care products are allowed to be labelled as organic even if only a very small percentage of the ingredients are organic. In organic processed food some non-organic ingredients may be allowed because they are not available in organic form.

Orthophenyl Phenol
Also known as E231 and OPP. Used in fresh produce packing industry as a preservative particularly for citrus fruit.

Ouzo

Greek alcoholic aperitif with a strong anise flavour.

Oxybenzone

Used in *sunscreens*, skin care and *lip balms*.

Ozone

Used in the treatment of *swimming pools*. As it dissipates rapidly, it cannot be used on its own, so some *chlorine* is generally used as well. Also a major form of *air pollution*. Not produced directly, but occurs as a result of sunlight acting on *nitrogen dioxide* and other chemicals in the air.

P

Packaging

Packaging can contaminate food and so may be an unsuspected cause of allergies. See *paper*, *phthalates*, *butylated hydroxytoluene* and *aluminium*.

Paint

The typical paint mixture is 5-25% pigment and 75-95% *solvent*. *Latex* paints and *acrylic* paints use water as the solvent. Other solvents used in paints include *naphtha*, *toluene*, and *xylene*. See also *water colour paints*.

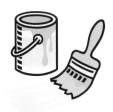

Palladium

Main exposure is through road dust where this metal is present from catalytic converters. Also used as a *dental* material and in electrical components. White gold is made from *gold* and palladium.

Palm Oil

Used to make *soap*, *polyurethanes*, polyacrylates, *glycerol*, *ghee*, *margarine* and *vegetable oil*. Also used in processed food.

Panthenol

Derived from vitamin B5. Found in moisturisers, hair conditioners, shampoos, hair sprays, *hair dyes*, *mascaras*, and after-shaves.

Papaya

A tropical fruit also known as paw paw.

Paper

Made from wood pulp, which is extracted from wood chippings, often using chemicals (*sodium hydroxide*, *sulphuric acid* or hydrogen sulphite). Most paper (for writing, printing, tea bags, coffee filters, paper towels etc.) is bleached using *chlorine* or *hydrogen peroxide*. China *clay* (or sometimes *calcium carbonate* or *titanium dioxide*) is used to increase the opacity of the paper for many applications. *Starch*, *rosin*, *aluminium sulphate*, *gelatine*, *latex* or synthetic compounds may be used to make the paper more water-repellent. *Silicon* powder is used to coat paper suitable for ink-jet printers. *Polyvinyl chloride* and *polyvinylidene chloride* may be used as a coating to increase the strength of the paper for *packaging*, etc. *Propyl gallate*, etc. may be used to coat paper that is indirect contact with food.

Parabens

A widely used group of preservatives in creams, *cosmetics*, food and beverages in the form of methyl, propyl, butyl and ethyl paraben. Typical products include hand creams, body lotions, tanning lotions, shampoos, skin cleansers, skin toners, moisturisers, hair conditioners, *hair dyes*, eye shadows, foundations and after-shaves.

Paradichlorobenzene

Used mainly as an insecticidal *fumigant* against clothes moths, and as an *air freshener*. Also used as an *insecticide* and *fungicide* on crops, and in the manufacture of *plastics*, *dyes* and *drugs*.

Paraffin

Also known as kerosene. Used in some heaters and furnaces, in hurricane lamps and jet engine fuel. Industrially used as a *solvent* for greases and *pesticides*. Also found in personal care products, hair creams, hand creams, and ointments. Various types used in ointments and creams (e.g. *paraffinum liquidum*, *white paraffin*, etc.) that have different properties (e.g. melting point) so are appropriate for different situations.

Paraffinum Liquidum

Also known as mineral oil jelly, petroleum jelly and petrolatum. A common component of *cosmetics*, personal care products and creams for *eczema* and *dermatitis*. See also *paraffin*.

Paraphenylenediamine (PPDA)

A chemical found in *hair dyes*, *elastic*, *shoes*, printers' ink and photographic developing agents. People with this sensitivity may also have problems with other dyes in dark clothing, especially when the fabric is man-made. May also react to some local *anaesthetics* that are chemically similar.

Parfum

In the USA the word 'fragrance' is used instead. Listed as an ingredient in *cosmetics*, personal care and household products. Can be natural or synthetic or a combination of both. Often a mixture of several different ones, and the exact proportions may vary over time depending on other smells in the product. May be used to give a perfume to a product, or to disguise the unpleasant smell of an active ingredient.

Parsley
In the same family as *carrot*.

Particulate Matter
Microscopic airborne particles. Two groups categorised according to size: PM10 and PM2.5. PM10 (less than 10 micrometres) particles originate from smoke, dirt and dust from industry, *vehicle exhaust fumes*, *pollens* and *moulds*. PM2.5 comes from heavy metals and toxic organic compounds produced by industry. PM2.5 can travel further than PM10 because they are lighter. Particles smaller than 10 micrometres can be inhaled, and almost everyone will have some of these particles in their lungs. Particles larger than 10 micrometers are usually sand and dirt blown by winds from roadways, fields, and construction sites.

Pasta
Usually made from *wheat*. May also contain *egg*, spinach, etc. Does not contain *baking powder*.

Patent Blue V
An artificial *food colouring* also known as E131, Food Blue 5 and C.I. 42051. Used in scotch eggs, and diagnostically to colour lymph vessels and veins. Banned in Australia, New Zealand USA and Norway.

Paw Paw
Also known as papaya.

PCBs
See *polychlorinated biphenols*.

Peanut

 A member of the legume family (along with peas, beans, lentils, etc.) rather than being a *nut* (but see page 146). Common allergen. Reactions can include *anaphylactic shock*. May be found in *vegetable oil*. *Arachis oil* is made from peanut oil. See also *aflatoxin*.

Pectin

A *stabiliser* also known as E440(a) or, when treated with *ammonia* known as E440(b). Commercially produced from rind of *citrus fruits* and *apples* that are a waste product from other manufacturing processes (e.g. *cider* making). Typical uses include in jam, jellies, confectionery, biscuits, yoghurt, desserts, *soft drinks*, salad dressings, dental *adhesives*, diarrhoea preparations and *cosmetics*. Naturally present in all plants.

Peeling Fruit And Vegetables

When fruit and vegetables are used in processed food, or frozen or canned, they often need to be peeled. This can be done either mechanically or using chemicals. Chemical peeling (also known as lye peeling), involves the use of *sodium hydroxide* (or sometimes *potassium hydroxide*) to loosen the skin, followed by strong water jets to remove the skin completely. The fruit or vegetable is then boiled briefly or washed with dilute *citric acid* to avoid it becoming discoloured through oxidation.

PEG

See *polyethylene glycol*.

PEG-20 Stearate

An emulsifier in *cosmetics*. See also *polyethylene glycol*.

PEG-100 Stearate
Used in personal care products, such as scrubs, masks and depilatory creams. See also *polyethylene glycol*.

Penicillin
The first group of *antibiotic* drugs to be discovered. Natural penicillins are derived from the mould penicillium. Other drugs are manufactured synthetically. People who are allergic to these drugs will often develop a rash when they take them. People who are sensitive are not necessarily also allergic to the mould *penicillium*.

Penicillium
A *mould*, commonly found on spoiled foods, compost heaps, *carpets*, wall paper, and in wine cellars. People who are sensitive are not necessarily also allergic to the antibiotic *penicillin*.

Penicillium Glaucum
The name of a mould responsible for the veining in some blue *cheeses*.

Penicillium Roqueforti
The name of a mould responsible for the veining in some blue *cheeses* (mainly but not only Roquefort).

Pentetate Pentasodium
Used in *hair dyes*, facial cleansers and *soap*.

Pepper (Black And White)

Pepper seems to be a problem for many people, particularly those suffering from various kinds of headaches.

PERC
See *perchloroethylene*.

Perchloroethylene

Also known as tetrachloroethylene, ethylene tetrachloride, or PERC. A *solvent* commonly used in *dry-cleaning* fluid, spot removers, *aerosols*, *shoe polishes* and typewriter correction fluid. Also used by car/automobile mechanics.

Perfume

Exposure to perfume occurs not only because of perfume the person uses themselves, but also those used by other people, and encountered in shops and household products. Easy to think of perfumes as only being used in perfumes, *air fresheners* and similar products, but perfumes (often a mixture of many different synthetic products) are
added to a whole range of products: *cosmetics*, personal care products, *detergents* and household cleaning agents, etc. The finished product will not necessarily have a strong smell, because the perfume may have been added to disguise the unpleasant smell of active ingredients, e.g. in *hair dyes*. Perfume mixes added to products known as *parfum* or *fragrance*. See also *unperfumed*.

Perfumed Products

See *perfume*, *parfum* and *unperfumed*.

Pernod

An anise-based alcoholic drink made in France.

Peroxide

See *hydrogen peroxide*.

Pesticides

 Chemicals used to kill insects, weeds, etc. Farm workers may have direct, intense contact with pesticides. The general population are also exposed to pesticide residues in food and pesticides travelling through the air from areas where they have been sprayed. May also be in drinking water, applied to road sides to control weeds, or used in some countries in public health programmes to control vectors, such as ticks that carry disease. Research has shown that pesticides that are long banned are still being encountered in food, water, etc. As well as the active ingredients there are also likely to be chemicals used to help the stickiness and consistency of the pesticide.

PET
See *polyethylene terephthalate*.

Pet Hair
See *pets* and *animal hair*.

Pets
Many people are allergic to pets. This does not necessarily happen immediately they own the pet. *Cats* are a particular problem, but other pets (*dogs*, hamsters, mice, gerbils, rats, rabbits, guinea pigs, horses, birds) may also be a problem. Children may also be exposed to pets at school. The urine of pet hamsters, mice, gerbils, rabbits and guinea pigs contains proteins that can trigger allergic reactions. Exposure is through contact with the living area of the pet. Also, when the urine dries, the proteins become airborne and can be inhaled, causing further problems. *Feathers* from birds may be a problem too. Dust and moulds from pet food and animal bedding may also affect some people. See also *dander*, *cat* and *dog*.

Petriella
Common indoor *mould* growing particularly on damp wood, so often found in bathrooms and in kitchens.

Petrol Exhaust Fumes
See *vehicle exhaust fumes*.

Petrolatum
See *paraffinum liquidum*.

Petroleum
See *crude oil*.

Petroleum Jelly
See *paraffinum liquidum*.

Pewter
A metal made predominantly of *tin*, with a small amount of another metal added (usually *antimony*, or *copper*). Britannia metal is a variety of pewter containing 96% tin and 4% antimony. Originally the additional metal was *lead*, but because of health concerns this is now not used. Used in decorative ware.

PG
See *propylene glycol*.

Pharmaceuticals
See *drugs*.

Phenethyl Alcohol
Used extensively in *perfumed products*.

Phenol
Also known as carbolic. One of the main constituents of man-made fibres such as *polyester* and *nylon*. Also used in the manufacture of *polyurethane*. A powerful disinfectant, so used in germicidal *soaps* and face washes, and as a preservative in medicines including injections and *vaccines*. Found in *pesticides*, *fungicides*, wood preservatives, floor levelling resins, hydraulic fluids and various industrial chemicals.

Phenolic Food Compounds

Also known as aromatic food compounds. Naturally found in plants and *pollens*, protecting plants against pathogens and aiding the dispersal and germination of seeds. Dr Darrell Weber, a plant chemist at the Brigham Young University in America, has found 13 different phenolics in *cow's milk*, 14 in *tomato* and 9 in *soya*. ('Journal of Orthomolecular Psychiatry' Vol 12, No 4). An allergy to several different foods could be a sensitivity to a phenolic food compound shared by these foods. Chemical structure of some of them very close to common allergens such as *phenol*, *benzene*, and *formaldehyde*.

Phenoxyethanol

Found in hair conditioners, sports body rubs, aqueous creams, skin toners, anti-bacterial and anti-fungal agents, *cosmetics* and *vaccines*.

Phenylenediamine

See paraphenylenediamine. When a reaction to *hair dye* occurs, this is the most likely culprit. Also in *cosmetics*, printing ink and *rubber* components.

Phenylmethanol

See *benzyl alcohol*.

Phenyl Methyl Acetate

See *benzyl acetate*.

Phoma

A fungus that is a common indoor allergen. Produces pink and purple spots on painted walls. May be found on *butter*, *paint*, *rubber* and *cement*.

Phosphoric Acid

Also known as E338. Used mainly in the production of agricultural fertilisers, but also used as an additive in *detergents*, for *insecticide* production, as a rust remover and in waste-water treatment. Typical food uses include in *soft drinks*, *beer* and cooked meats. Also used in hair lightening cream.

Photocopiers

The machines produce *ozone*. The toner is a mixture of *plastic* particles (e.g. *styrene acrylate copolymer* or *polypropylene*), *iron oxide* and pigments (e.g. *carbon black*) and *paraffin* wax.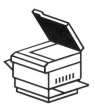

Phthalates

A group of chemicals that help to make *plastics* soft. Have been shown to migrate from plastic packaging into food. Common ones are bis(2-ethylhexyl) phthalate and *dioctyl phthalate*.

Pillows

Pillows can be made from different materials, e.g. *polyester*, *polyurethane* foam, *latex* and *feathers*.

Pine Oil

Derived from steam distillation of wood from pine trees. A common agent used in many household disinfectants and deodorants.

Plants

Some plants cause irritation from their sap, but allergic reactions can also occur to any plant. Common culprits include marigolds, ivy (especially *poison ivy*), dandelions, daffodils, tulips, hydrangeas and primroses. Plants, particularly house plants, often harbour *moulds*. See also *pollens, grass, flower pollens* and *tree pollens*.

Plastics
There are hundreds of different types of plastics, e.g. *polyethylene, polyvinyl chloride, polycarbonate*, etc. Different plastics have different qualities, (e.g. strength, flexibility, resistance to heat, etc.), so are suitable for different applications. See also *plasticisers*.

Plasticisers
Chemicals (often *phthalates*) that help to make *plastics* soft and pliable. Can migrate into the food from the plastic wrapping.

Platinum
Found in road dust from catalytic converters, high quality glassware, *dental* alloys, anti-cancer drugs, jewellery, computer hard disks and other electronic components. Photographic workers and workers in metal refineries may have problems with platinum salts.

Poison Ivy /Oak/Sumach
Three related plants that contain the oil urushiol. A problem in the USA and parts of Canada. The usual reaction is itching and small blisters in susceptible people.

Polenta
Derived from *corn* meal and used in Italian and African cookery.

Pollens
The amount of pollen in the air is closely related to the weather. Pollen counts are low on cold, rainy days and high on hot dry days. Prevailing winds will also affect the concentration of pollens in a given area. Highest pollen counts occur in morning and late afternoon in the immediate vicinity of the plants, but will be later if the pollen is carried on the wind to an area.

Pollen problems start much earlier in the year than many people think. In England, for example, the first pollens are around in February and March (some garden flowers and gorse). Then *tree pollens* are mainly from March to May, grass pollens are prominent in June and July, and weed pollens come into their own in July, August and September. See Appendix 3 for an international pollen calendar. So it is possible to have symptoms starting very early in the year and lasting into late summer, although most people will react to a more limited range of pollens.

Traditionally associated with *hay fever* and *asthma*, but in my experience they can contribute to many other problems as well. Many people are not aware that pollens affect them: they think they have just got a cold. In conversation they will admit that summer colds are much worse than winter ones because they last so long. When I show them that they are sensitive to pollens, they are amazed, because they have assumed that hay fever involves sneezing, itchy eyes etc. See also *flower pollens*, *tree pollens* and *grass*.

Pollution

The main outdoor air pollutants are *sulphur dioxide, nitrogen dioxide, ozone, carbon monoxide* and *particulate matter*. Many of the chemicals that are released by industrial processes into the air travel thousands of miles, and so the effect can be felt in rural as well as urban areas, and in urban areas that do not have 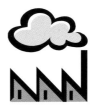 those particular types of industries. At first sight most people appear to have very little contact with some chemicals (e.g. *vinyl chloride*), because they are not used directly in consumer goods, but there are low levels in the air even many miles from where they are being used in manufacturing processes. See also *particulate matter* and page 10.

Polybrominated Diphenyl Ethers

Also known as PBDEs. A flame retardant found in foam furniture padding and other textiles, as well as the hard *plastics* used to house electronic equipment, including computers. Significant levels have been found as a contaminant in breast milk.

Polycarbonate

An unbreakable and shatterproof *plastic*. Used for food and beverage containers, baby bottles, water cooler bottles, and milk bottles. Also used for windows in greenhouses and conservatories, medical equipment, household appliances, CD's and DVD's. Also used in lightweight lenses in spectacles, helmets and visors. See also *bisphenol A*.

Polychlorinated Biphenols

Also known as PCB's. A group of chemicals that contain 209 individual compounds. Banned in the 1970's but still found in the environment, electrical equipment, wall coverings, *paints* and *plastic*. Have been found in *breast milk*.

Polyester

Also known by the trade names of Dacron and Trevira. Used in clothing, home furnishing, hoses, power belting, ropes, nets, thread, tyres, cord, sails, toothbrush bristles and upholstery in cars. Also used as a soft filling material for various products including *pillows*, *bedding* and furniture.

Polyethylene

Also known as polythene. The most widely used *plastic*. Two types: high-density polyethylene and low-density polyethylene. Used to make children's toys, carrier bags, bin liners and industrial bags, Also used extensively for consumer packaging including shrink film and squeezy bottles for food, personal care products, etc.. Also found as *carpet* backing and in *joint replacements*.

Polyethylene Glycol

Also known as PEG. Typical products include oven cleaner, personal care products, *cosmetics*, medicinal ointments, *capsules* and suppositories, and *detergents*. See also *PEG-20 stearate* and *PEG-100 stearate*.

Polyethylene Terephthalate

Also known as PET. A *plastic* that is used to make disposable drink bottles, oven ready meal trays, audio tapes, insulation in clothing and carpeting, filling for *pillows* and sleeping bags, etc.

Polyglycerol Esters Of Fatty Acids

An *emulsifier* also known as E475. Used in desserts and cake icing/frosting.

Polyglycerol Polyricinoleate

An *emulsifier* also known as E476. Used in desserts and cake icing/frosting.

Polyisobutylene

See *butyl rubber*.

Polypropylene

A *plastic* used for dishwasher-safe and microwavable food containers, yoghurt pots and margarine tubs, confectionery and tobacco packaging. Used for *carpets* under the trade names of Olefin, Astra, Zylon and Charisma. Other uses include toys, drinking straws, car/automobile interiors, artificial grass, bristles for brushes and brooms, thermal and cold weather sports clothing, and toner for *photocopiers* and printers.

Polysorbate 20

Also known as E432. Derived from *sorbitol*, and used widely in *cosmetics*.

Polysorbate 80

Also known as E433. An *emulsifier*, used in medicinal *tablets*, personal care products and some foods, e.g. *ice cream*.

Polystyrene

Probably the second most common *plastic* after *polyethylene*. Used for hot food and drink containers, plastic cutlery, packing material including egg cartons, the housing of computers, radios and household appliances, car/automobile interiors, low-cost toys, buoyancy aids, domestic water softening systems and *cavity wall insulation*.

Polytetrafluoroethylene

Also known as PTFE and Teflon. Used in non-stick cookware, plumbers' jointing tape, and as an additive in lubricants.

Polythene

See *polyethylene*.

Polyurethane

Found in *paints*, *varnishes*, foamed *plastics* for insulation, cushions, *mattresses, carpet* underlay, upholstery and in the building industry. Also used as an alternative to plaster casts for broken limbs. Used to make *elastane*.

Polyvinyl Acetate Phthalate

Used as a coating on *drugs*.

Polyvinyl Chloride

Also known as PVC. Typical uses include raincoats, car/automobile interiors, furnishings (as mock leather), food wrappings (becoming less common), plastic bottles for drinks and personal care products, coatings for *paper*, *shoe* soles, plastic pipes and building materials. In hospitals also used for catheters, blood bags and tubing.

Polyvinyl Pyrrolidone

Also known as PVP. Found in *adhesives*, personal care products, hair sprays, *detergents*, and drugs. Also used in *textile* industry for fibre treatment, and in ink for ink jet *printers* (helps *paper* and ink bond together more effectively).

Poly(vinylidene Chloride)

Also known as PVDC. Used as plastic wrapping for foods, and finishes on some *paper*.

Ponceau 4R

A *food colouring*, also known as E124, Cochineal Red, Food Red 7 and C.I. 16255. Typical uses include in soups, salami, seafood dressings, confectionery, desserts and *drugs*. Banned in some countries.

Poppadums

Served with Indian food. Can contain lentil flour, rice flour, *sodium bicarbonate* and spices.

Pork

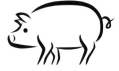

Ham and bacon are derived from *pork*. *Lard* is made from pork fat.

Potassium Benzoate

Also known as E212. A preservative. Typical products include *margarine*, pickles, prepared salad, fruit juice and *soft drinks*. Now being used increasingly in place of *sodium benzoate* because of its low sodium content.

Potassium Dichromate

Used in *cement*, *leather* tanning, safety matches, *paints* (especially anti-rust paints), *adhesives*, pigments, *detergents* and wood ash.

Potassium Hexacyanoferrate (II) Trihydrate

Also known as potassium ferrocyanide, YPP and E536. Used as an *anti-caking agent* in salt.

Potassium Hydrogen Tartrate

See *cream of tartar*.

Potassium Hydroxide

Food uses include washing or chemical *peeling of fruit and vegetables*, poultry preparation (to loosen feathers), and in cocoa processing. Also used in the production of pretzels, *soft drinks*, *ice cream* and *drugs*. May also be used in *detergents*, denture cleaners and drain cleaners.

Potassium Permanganate

Used in the treatment of water to remove iron, manganese, *hydrogen sulphide*, taste and odour.

Potassium Sorbate

A food preservative also known as E202. Used in *soft drinks*, *wines*, salad dressings and dips, ready-prepared sandwiches, *cakes* and desserts.

Potassium Stearate
Used as a thickener in personal care products, such as cleansing lotions and shampoos.

Potato
Part of an extensive botanical family including tomatoes, chilli, (bell) peppers and tobacco. Modified potato starch is used in sweet as well as savoury products. See also *acryalmide*.

Praline
Confectionery including *nuts*. Depending on the place this could be pecans in New Orleans, USA, or almonds/ hazelnuts in Europe.

Prawn
Some people are allergic to a muscle protein found in prawns and *shrimps* and *house dust mite*. If a prawn sensitivity is caused by this protein, the person will also react to shrimp and house dust mite. A common cause of *anaphylactic shock* and other extreme allergic reactions.

Printers
See *photocopiers*.

Printing
See *paper* and *newsprint*.

Processing Agents
See *accidental contaminants*.

Propane
A by-product of *petroleum* refining. Used as a propellant in hair spray. Also used as a fuel in gas-fired barbecues, portable lamps, agricultural and industrial heating and drying, on-site asphalt production, etc.

Propyl Gallate

Also known as E310. An *antioxidant* used in sausages, *margarine, chewing gum*, personal care products and *cosmetics*. Used in manufacture of *paper packaging* that will be in contact with food.

Propylene Glycol

Also known as PG, and propan-1,2-diol, and propylenglycolum. Used as an anti-freeze, a *solvent* and a mould inhibitor. Also used in the preparation of *perfumes*, in personal care products (e.g. cleansers, skin creams, *toothpastes*, shampoos, hair conditioners, *hair dyes*), and *cosmetics*, and in *drugs*. Used as a preservative in some food (e.g. *ice cream* and sour cream). Also used in artificial smoke or fog machines.

Propyl Paraben

See *parabens*.

PVC

See *polyvinyl chloride*.

PVP

See *polyvinyl pyrrolidone*.

Q

Quaternium-15

Preservative in *cosmetics*, personal care products, and household polishes and cleaners.

Quinoa

Used as though a *grain*, but is the seeds of a plant that is distantly related to spinach.

Quinoline Yellow

A *food colouring*, also known as E104, Food Yellow 13 and C.I. 470005. Typical uses include confectionery and *soft drinks*. Banned in Japan, Norway and the United States.

R

Rabbit

Rabbit hair is a common allergen in those exposed to it. Children may encounter rabbits at school as well as at home. Angora wool comes from rabbit.

Rapeseed

Known as canola in America. The oil is widely used in processed foods, *vegetable oils* and *margarine*. The *pollen* seems to be a particular problem in the UK (flowering in May).

Ragweed

Ragweed is a major problem in North America, in late summer and early autumn, causing *hay fever* type symptoms. In Europe only found in the French Rhône valley and some areas of Eastern Europe.

Most ragweed allergy problems caused by Ambrosia artemisiifolia (short or normal ragweed) and Ambrosia trifida (giant ragweed). Ragweed pollen can travel over 400 miles. Melon, *banana*, chamomile and sunflower seeds share some of the same chemicals. Marsh elder and mugwort pollen closely related botanically.

Raisins
Dried *grapes*.

Ramie
Made from Chinese grass or rhea, a plant with fibrous leaves. Used with other fibres as a blend in fabrics resembling *linen*.

Raw Food
See *cooked food*.

Rayon
Originally named as artificial silk. A fabric made from *cellulose*. Several different types depending on the chemicals that are used in the processing. Main type in use now is viscose rayon, sometimes just called viscose. Found in clothing, furnishings, *carpets* and feminine hygiene products such as *tampons*.

Red 2G
A *food colouring*, also known as E128 and C.I. 18050. A red synthetic dye found mainly in cooked meat products and sausages but can also be found in jams and drinks. Britain is the only European Union country to allow Red 2G. Banned in Australia, New Zealand, Canada, Japan, Norway, and the United States.

Red Wine
See *wine*.

Rennin
See *chymosin*.

Rennet

A natural extract from the stomach of calves used to make *cheese*. Cheese suitable for vegetarians does not use animal rennet, but usually uses a fungus (Mucor miehei) or sometimes a bacteria (Bacillus subtilis or Bacillus prodigiosum). May also be produced from genetically modified sources.

Resin

Can be either natural or synthetic. Natural resins come from various plants and trees. Used in *varnishes* and *lacquers*. See also *colophony* and *shellac*

Resorcin

See *resorcinol*.

Resorcinol

Also known as resorcin. Used to treat acne and skin complaints. Also used in *hair dyes*, wood *adhesives*, UV blocking preparations, *cosmetics*, and to *dye* fur and *leather*.

Riboflavin

Also known as Vitamin B2 and E101. A *natural food colouring* used in sauces, processed *cheese*, dairy products, desserts, baby food, breakfast cereals and *soft drinks*. Also used as a vitamin supplement.

Rice

Rice bran wax may be found in *chewing gum* as plasticising material.

Rosin

See *colophony*.

Rubber

Either natural (see *latex*) or synthetic (made from *crude oil*). Synthetic rubber is used more extensively than natural rubber. There are various types of synthetic rubber including styrene-butadiene, polybutadiene, *butyl rubber*, *nitrile*, etc.

Rubber Gloves

Made from various materials including *latex*, *nitrile*, *polyurethane* and *polyvinyl chloride*. Small amounts of *chalk* may be present on new gloves (used as a releasing agent in manufacturing). Corn starch used so that thin latex gloves are easier to put on.

Rum

An alcoholic drink made from fermented and distilled *molasses*.

Rust

See *iron oxide*.

Rye

A grain containing some *gluten*. *Bread* sold as rye bread may contain *wheat* to help it rise. Used in Canadian and American *whiskey*.

S

Saccharin

An artificial sweetener commonly found in *soft drinks*, low-calorie foods and *toothpastes*.

Salicylate

This chemical occurs naturally in some foods, particularly dried apricots, dates, raisins, gherkins and many herbs and spices. *Aspirin* (and some other *drugs*) contains acetyl salicylic acid and many people are allergic to this. May or may not also be allergic to naturally occurring salicylates. Bruised fruit and vegetables also contain higher levels of salicylates than their unbruised counterparts. Individuals with salicylate sensitivity will often also react to preservatives, particularly *sodium benzoate* and *potassium benzoate*, and the *food colouring tartrazine*.

Salicylic Acid

Used as a preservative and antiseptic in personal care products. May be a residue in *milk* from use with dairy animals.

Salt

Cooking and table salt, and salt used in processed foods often contains *anti-caking agents* to help it flow more freely. Potassium iodide is added to salt to make iodised table salt. *Sugar*, *sodium bicarbonate*, *sodium carbonate*, or sodium thiosulfate may be used to stabilise the potassium iodide. See also *sodium chloride*.

Semen

Some people are allergic to their partner's semen, and this can hinder conception. This is most likely to be to a protein produced by the prostate, but it could also be a reaction to traces of *drugs* or food eaten by the man and found in his semen. The reaction may be localised to the areas exposed to the semen, or may involve a more generalised reaction including skin irritation or breathing problems.

Semolina

A form of *wheat*.

Sheep Dip
Used by sheep farmers. Organo-phosphates (e.g. diazinon and propetamphos) were used solely until the early 1990's when synthetic pyrethroids (e.g. cypermethrin and flumethrin) were introduced.

Sheep's Milk
Those who are allergic to *cow's milk* may also be allergic to sheep's milk, although not necessarily on first exposure.

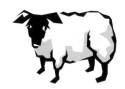

Sheep's Wool
See *wool*.

Shellac
Also known as 904 (no E). Derived from insects. Used to coat food and tablets, and also used in some *varnishes* and *paints*.

Sherry
A *wine* fortified with *brandy*.

Shoes
See *footwear*.

Shoe Polishes

Usually contains chemicals such as *trichloroethylene*, ethylene glycol, *methylene chloride*, *nitrobenzene*, *turpentine* and *carbon black*. Gel polishes may contain *carageenan*.

Shrimp
Some people are allergic to a muscle protein found in shrimp that is also found in *prawn* and *house dust mite*.

Silicones

Used widely as water repellent *adhesives* and sealers. Used as lubricants in many industries including food manufacturing. Silicone anti-foam may be used to minimise unwanted foam during food and drink processing for *fruit juices*, tofu, freeze-dried *coffee*, snack foods and *wine*. Used in medicinal creams and gels, personal care products, *cosmetics*, *paints* and inks.

Silk Amino Acids

Derived from silk and used in *cosmetics* and personal care products.

Silver

A metal found in *dental amalgam*, jewellery, some *water filters* and electrical components. Also used as a *food colouring* (E174) but solely for external decoration. 'Silver' *coins* do not usually contain silver because of its cost.

SLS

See *sodium lauryl sulphate*.

Smoked Food

Some smoked food has colouring (typically E154, also known as brown FK, and kipper brown) and flavourings added.

Soap

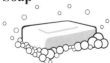 Basic ingredients are *tallow*, *coconut* oil and *palm oil*, plus *perfumes*, and often chemicals to increase foaming, act as preservatives or as *surfactants*, etc. *Sodium hydroxide* used in its preparation, but appears to be absent from the finished product, as it is used up in the chemical reactions that take place. See also *liquid soap*.

Soda Ash

See *sodium carbonate*.

Sodium Alginate
Also known as E401. A *stabiliser* used in cakes, desserts, *ice cream*, cereal bars, and *fruit juices*. Also used to stabilise the foam on *beer*.

Sodium Aluminium Phosphate
Also known as E541. A raising agent used as one of the ingredients in *baking powder*.

Sodium Benzoate
A food preservative also known as E211. Typical products include *soft drinks*, salad dressings, barbecue sauces, and *margarine*. Also used in personal care products (such as body washes, shampoos and mouth washes) and in many oral *drugs*.

Sodium Bicarbonate

Also known as baking soda, bicarbonate of soda, sodium hydrogen carbonate and E500. Used in *baked goods, poppadums*. Used as a source of carbon dioxide in some *soft drinks*. Used to treat *wool* and silk, and in dyeing and printing fabrics. Widely used in the *rubber* and *plastics* industry as a blowing agent, and also in waste water treatment. Also produced by the body in the pancreatic juices.

Sodium Bisulphite
See *sodium hydrogen sulphite*.

Sodium Carbonate
Also known as soda ash. The active ingredient in washing soda. Used in the production of glass, *soap*, *detergents*, *paper* and *textiles*.

Sodium Carboxy Methylcellulose
Also known as E466 and carboxymethyl cellulose. A thickener often found in *ice cream*, cakes, puddings, *soft drinks*, *toothpastes*

and some *drug tablets*. Also used in *detergents* to stop grime reattaching to *fabrics*.

Sodium Caseinate
Made from *cow's milk*, using *sodium hydroxide.* May be added to cereals and *baked goods* to increase their nutrient value. Used as a *stabiliser* in milk shakes and diabetic *ice cream*, as a binder in meat products such as sausages, meat loaves and luncheon meat, and as a clarifier in *wine* production. May also be found in *coffee creamers*, and cottage cheese.

Sodium Chloride
Also known as *salt*. Used in *soap,* skin and hair preparations, as well as in processed food.

Sodium Citrate
Used as an acidity regulator in food and beverages. Commonly found in jams, jellies, desserts, *soft drinks*, confectionery and shampoo.

Sodium Hexacyanoferrate (II) Decahydrate
Also known as sodium ferrocyanide, yellow prussiate of soda, YPS and E535. An *anti-caking agent* used in salt.

Sodium Hexametaphosphate
A chemical used in frozen fish to inhibit moisture loss on defrosting. Also used in industrial water treatment, and in textile dyeing.

Sodium Hydrogen Carbonate
See *sodium bicarbonate*.

Sodium Hydrogen Sulphite
Also known as E222, sodium bisulphite and acid sodium sulphite. A preservative used in food, such as instant potato mixes and *soft drinks*.

Sodium Hydroxide
Also known as caustic soda. Used in the production of *soap*, *detergents*, *paper* and *aluminium*. Many other chemicals are made from it. Also used in the commercial *peeling of fruit and vegetables*. Used in the preparation of some foods (e.g. Norwegian lutefish, pretzels, hominy grits and some olives). Also found in oven cleaners and furniture-stripping dips.

Sodium Hypochlorite
The active ingredient in household *bleach* (chlorine bleach). Used in household disinfectants, water purifiers, treatment of drinking *water* and *swimming pool* water, sewage treatment, and chemical toilets. Also may be used in manufacture of *denim* cloth to give a faded look.

Sodium Laureth Sulphate
A common chemical in personal care products, such as shampoos, hair conditioners, *hair dyes*, shower gels, body washes, and baby bath liquids.

Sodium Lauryl Sulphate
Also known as SLS. Used to create foam, suds or a creamy texture in a wide range of products, e.g. *toothpastes*, shampoos, hair conditioners, body washes, shaving creams, denture cleaners and *detergents*.

Sodium Metabisulphate
A food preservative also known as E223. Typical product uses include pre-squeezed lemon juice, pickles, prepared salad, *soft drinks* and alcoholic drinks.

Sodium Nitrate

Also known as E251. Used as a preservative in processed meat products such as sausages, bacon and ham, as well as artificially smoked fish.

Sodium Nitrite

Also known as E250. A preservative used in meat products.

Sodium Perborate

Used in *detergents* as a bleaching agent.

Sodium Silicate

Added to *detergents* and *dishwasher powders* to prevent corrosion of the machine by the active ingredients in the powder.

Sodium Stearoyl Lactylate

Used as a dough strengthener in baked products, and as a *stabiliser* in icings/frostings, fillings, puddings, tea and *coffee creamers*. Also found in dehydrated potato, snack dips and cheese.

Sodium Stearyl Fumarate

Found in medicinal *tablets*, and also used as a dough conditioner in commercial *bread* making.

Sodium Tripolyphosphate

Also known as E450(b). Used as an *emulsifier* in meat products and processed cheese. Also used in *detergents*, *dishwasher powders* and household and industrial cleaners.

Soft Drinks

Manufacturers may or may not use municipal *water* supply. Almost always subjected to additional treatments. Contain a variety of ingredients that may include *sugar*, *glucose*, *artificial sweeteners*, *caffeine*, *food colourings, flavouring, stabilisers, phosphoric acid, ascorbic acid, potassium benzoate*, etc.

Solvents
Widely used industrially both in the actual production process and in cleaning agents. Used in the food industry in extraction processes to maximise the amount extracted, so used in the production of *fruit juices, vegetable oils, natural food colours*, herbal preparations, etc. Also used to disperse substances in solution or in suspension, so that they can be better integrated into a product (foods, confectionery, cosmetics and personal care products). Small quantities will remain in the finished product. See *carry over ingredients*.

Sorbic Acid
Also known as E200. Uses include in medicinal *tablets, cosmetics*, cheese, syrups, *soft drinks* and *adhesives*.

Sorbitan Monostearate
An emulsifier also known as E491. Used in dried *yeast*, cakes, desserts, *baked goods*, imitation whipped cream, liquid tea concentrates, haemorrhoid cream and cream for dry skin.

Sorbitol
Also known as E420. Used as a sweetener and to preserve the moisture content in food and confectionery. Also used in diabetic and low-calorie foods. Commonly found in *toothpastes*, face wash creams, medicinal syrups and cough mixtures. Involved in the manufacture of *ascorbic acid*. Naturally present in rowan berries. See also *polysorbate 20* and *polysorbate 80*.

Soy
See *soya*.

Soya

A member of the bean family used to make *meat substitutes*, tofu, soya sauce, miso, tempeh and soya milk. Also used to make *vegetable oil*, *vitamin* E, *lecithin*, and found in some *newsprint*.

Soy(a) Lecithin

See *lecithin*.

Spandex

See *elastane*.

Spelt

One of the first *grains* to be grown by our ancestors when they started to cultivate the land. Distantly related to *wheat*, but can often be tolerated when wheat cannot be. Used in Italy under the name of faro, and also in central Europe.

Stabilisers

Chemicals added to products to stop the ingredients from separating out. Can be used industrially, and in the production of food, beverages, personal care products and *cosmetics*.

Stachybotrys

A common indoor black *mould*, particularly in areas of high humidity that experience temperature fluctuations.

Stainless Steel

A hard-wearing rust-resistant alloy of *iron*, *chromium* and *nickel*. Widely used in the home, in industry, hospitals and in food processing. Specific uses include for *joint replacements*, some *coins*, *cutlery*, cooking utensils, etc.

Stamps

The glue is usually made from *gum Arabic*, *gum tragacanth* or *tapioca* starch.

Starch

This can come from a grain (e.g. *wheat* or *corn*) or from vegetables. See *modified starch* and *inulin*.

Steareth

A family of chemicals (e.g. steareth-2, steareth-100). Used in *hair dyes* and lightening preparations, and other personal care products.

Stearic Acid

A chemical found in personal care products (e.g. moisturisers, hand creams, body lotions, tanning lotions, cream soaps, eye shadows, *mascaras*, *hair dyes*, foundation, and shaving foams). Used as a lubricant in nutritional and medicinal *tablets*.

Stearyl Ether

Found in personal care products.

Steel

Made from *iron* and carbon. See *stainless steel*.

Sterculia Gum

See *gum karaya*.

Stoddard solvent

Used as a paint thinner. Found in some types of *photocopier* toners, printing inks, and *adhesives*. Also used as a *dry cleaning solvent*, and as a general cleaner and degreaser.

Storage Mite

Storage mites in hay and grain are often the culprits for farmers rather than the hay or grain itself. People who react to these often also allergic to *house dust mite*.

Styrene
Also known as ethenylbenzene, vinylbenzene and butadiene.
Involved in manufacture of *polystyrene* and synthetic *rubber*. Used
in composite *dental fillings*, floor waxes, *paints*, *adhesives*
(including those for artificial nails), putty, metal cleaners and
car/automobile body fillers. Also found in *tobacco smoke*.

Styrene Acrylate Copolymer
Found in toner for *photocopiers* and printers, primer sealers, and
some personal care products.

Sucrose
The chemical name for *sugar*.

Sugar
Also known as sucrose. The most widely used sugar is derived from
either cane or beet sugar. Some people will react regardless of the
origins of the sugar. Others will only react to one type, which is not
surprising when you consider that cane is a member of the *grain*
botanical family and beet is a member of the family that includes
spinach and chard. One client could not understand her fluctuating
symptoms till we identified that sometimes she was buying cane
sugar and sometimes beet sugar to put into her cups of tea, and she
was only allergic to one type.

Manufactured goods will often just list 'sugar' as an ingredient,
because manufacturers will use the cheapest sugar available at the
time, so the product may contain beet sugar on one occasion and
cane sugar on another. Found in a whole range of processed foods
including savoury ones. Also see *dextrose*, *fructose* and *glucose*.

Sulphur Dioxide
Also known as E220. A preservative found in dried fruit, desiccated
coconut, fruit pie fillings, sausage meat, potato products, relishes,
wine and *beer*.

Sulphuric Acid
Involved in *paper, plastic, detergent* and fertiliser production. Also in the manufacture of *titanium dioxide* and other pigments.

Sultana
A type of *raisin*, but from only one variety of grape (the green, seedless Sultana grape).

Sunflower Seeds
Used in some *vegetable oils*, speciality *breads*, muesli, etc. The oil may be used in nutritional capsules where the nutrients are suspended in oil.

Sunscreen Preparations

Contain various ingredients including *octyl methoxycinnamate*, octyl salicitate, *oxybenzone*, *titanium dioxide*, trimethylsiloxysilicate. See also *sun tan preparations*.

Sunset Yellow
An orange *food colouring* also known as E110, Orange Yellow 5, FD & C Yellow No. 6, Food Yellow 3 and C.I. 15985. Widely used in the food industry (e.g. cereals, *baked goods*, snack foods, jams and marmalade, *ice cream*, desserts, confectionery and *soft drinks*). Also used in *cosmetics* and *drugs*. Banned in Finland and Norway.

Sun Tan Preparations (Fake Tanning Products)
These fake tan preparations contain a variety of chemicals. The most important one is *dihydroxyacetone*. See also *sunscreen preparations*.

Surfactants

Chemicals (e.g. sodium cholate and lauryldimethylamine-oxide) added to aid the mixing of ingredients, by lowering the surface tension of the liquid. Used in fabric dyeing, detergents, personal care products, etc.

Surfecants

See *surfactants*.

Surgical Sutures

Generally made from man-made materials (such as *polyethylene terephthalate*, *polypropylene*, polydioxanone and polyglycolic acid), and occasionally silk. Dissolvable sutures usually made from *collagen* (mainly from beef and/or sheep).

Swimming Pool Water

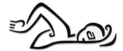 *Chlorine* on its own, or with *ozone*, is the main treatment. Many people are aware of reacting to swimming pool water. Common symptoms include *rashes*, *headaches*, sore and itchy eyes, nose and throats. Often assumed that it is the chlorine in the water that is causing the problem, but other chemicals may be involved (e.g. *bromine*). *Aluminium* coagulants may be used to aid the treatment of swimming pool water. Also organisms such as E. coli and the parasite cryptosporidium and giardia can occasionally be found in badly maintained swimming pools. Even in well-maintained pools there will be traces of urea, dead skin cells and human waste in the water. Chemicals interacting with these can produce other chemicals such as *trihalomethanes*.

T

Tablets

Many tablets contain synthetic *colourings*, or have information stamped on them in ink, so that different strengths or composition are more evident to minimise dispensing errors. Will also include 'inactive' ingredients to aid in the manufacture and increase ease of use. Includes *corn* starch, *lactose*, silica, polyvidone, *polysorbate 80*, *talc*, *magnesium stearate*, magnesium hydroxide, *aluminium silicate*, *paraffin*, various forms of *cellulose*, *stearic acid*, *titanium dioxide*
carnauba wax, agar, etc. Usually more inactive ingredients than *capsules*. See also *drugs*, *nutritional supplements* and *herbal supplements*.

Tabletting Agent

See *tablets*.

TAED

See *tetra acetyl ethylene diamine*.

Talc

Also known as magnesium silicate hydroxide. Primary ingredient in talcum powder. Also found in medicinal *tablets*, and used as a filler material for *paints*, *rubber* and *insecticides*.

Tallow

Made from animal fats. Used in solid *soap*.

Tampons

Made from *rayon* and/or *cotton*. Chemicals are usually used to clean and whiten the fibres during manufacture.

Tannic Acid

See *tannin*.

Tannin

Derived commercially from oak bark and used in tanning *leather* and to fix *dyes* in *textile* manufacture. Used in production of red *wine*. Also present in *tea*.

Tapioca

Derived from the plant cassava. Used as a flour in some desserts and *baked goods*. Converted into modified *starch* for use in processed foods. Also used for the glue for *stamps* and *envelopes*, and in industrial processes making *monosodium glutamate*, *antibiotics*, etc. Use increasing.

Tap Water

See *water*.

Tartaric Acid

Also known as E334. Commonly found in *baking powder* and jams. Also used in printing and in photographic developing.

Tartrazine

Also known as E102, FD & C Yellow No 5, Food Yellow 4 and C.I. 19140. A widely used yellow-orange *food colouring*. Used with Brilliant Blue FCF to produce various green shades. Typical products include *soft drinks*, *ice cream*, confectionery and *baked goods*. Used extensively in *perfume*, skin care, *cosmetics* and *drugs*.

Tattoo Dyes

Most tattoo dyes come from metals, such as *iron*, *mercury*, *cadmium*, *chromium*, *cobalt*, *manganese*, *zinc*, *lead*, and *titanium*. The dyes may also contain resin, *acrylic* and *glycol*.

Tea

Tea bags contain bleaches and *adhesives*. See also *decaffeination* and *tannin*.

TEA
See *triethanolamine*.

Teflon
See *polytetrafluoroethylene*.

Terpenes
A group of chemicals derived from plants. Best known ones are *pine oil*, *turpentine*, and camphor oil.

Terpineol
A widely used fragrance in *perfumed products*.

Tetra Acetyl Ethylene Diamine
Also known as TAED. A *bleach* activator used in *detergents*, cleaners and in *paper*-making.

Tetrachloroethylene
See *perchloroethylene*.

Textiles
See *fabrics*.

Thai Fish Sauce
Also known as nam pla. A fermentation of small, whole fish (sometimes *shrimps*). Used extensively in Vietnamese and Thai cooking.

Theobromine
A stimulant found naturally in *tea*, *coffee*, *cola* and *chocolate*.

Theophylline
A stimulant found naturally in *tea*, *coffee*, *cola* and *chocolate*.

Thimerosal
A *mercury* compound, used as a preservative in contact lens solutions, injectable drugs, *vaccines* and *cosmetics*.

Thiuram
A chemical mixture found in *rubber* gloves and boots, *shoes*, rubber handles, rubber kitchen utensils, balloons, *condoms*, *elastic*, *insecticides*, *fungicides*, disinfectants and seed dressings.

Timothy Grass
A common allergen. In the UK it flowers from June to August. See also *grass*.

Tin
A metal found in *dental amalgam*, canning, and solder in iron and copper pipes. Compounds used in *fungicides* and glass coatings. Small quantities in some *coins*. *Bronze* contains some tin. Main ingredient in *pewter*.

Titanium
A metal used in *dental* work, *joint replacements*, and jewellery.

Titanium Dioxide
Also known as E171 and C.I. 77891. A *food colouring* used in confectionery, sauces, desserts, *toothpastes*, *sunscreens*, *gelatine capsules*, *tablets*, *lipsticks*, foundation, *mascaras*, *nail polishes*, *paint* pigments, printing ink, art materials, filler for *paper* and *plastics*. In confectionery often used to provide a barrier between different colours. Banned in Germany.

Toast

When *bread* is toasted, it produces vegetable charcoal. Some people react to this, but are perfectly fine with the untoasted bread.

Tobacco Smoke

Many people are allergic to tobacco smoke, and can be affected even when they do not smoke themselves. Contains many different chemicals including *benzene, formaldehyde, styrene, nicotine, cotinine* and *carbon monoxide.* See also *cigarettes* and *cigarette filters.*

Tocopherol Acetate

Found in face wash creams, hair conditioners, hand creams, foundation, eye shadows, *lipsticks*, and similar products.

Toluene

A high-octane aviation and motor fuel. Used in the manufacture of *benzene*, caprolactam, *phenol* and *dyes*. Found in damp treatments, *adhesives*, inks, *paints*, lacquers, *perfumes*, *nail polish*, furniture polish, degreasers and cleaners.

Tomato

In the same botanical family as *potato*. Widely used in processed foods.

Toothpaste

Common abrasives include calcium phosphates, *calcium carbonate*, and silica. If the toothpaste contains fluoride, it will be in the form of sodium monofluorophosphate, stannous fluoride, or sodium fluoride. Foaming agent is often *sodium*

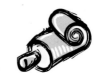

lauryl sulphate. Glycerin and *sorbitol* are used to stop the toothpaste drying out. *Carrageenan* and *xanthan gum* are common thickening agents. *Sodium benzoate* and *parabens* used as preservatives. *Food colourings*, *flavourings* and *artificial sweeteners* are also likely to be added.

Toxicity
Unfortunately there are many toxic chemicals in the modern environment – some of them are listed in this book. If people are allergic to one of these toxic chemicals, they are even less able to counteract it. In consequence they are likely to find exposure to lower levels of these toxic chemicals difficult to cope with.

Treacle
See *molasses*.

Tree Pollens
The most allergenic tree *pollens* vary according to region, but may include oak, birch, elder and olive. See also *pollens*, *flower pollens* and appendix 3.

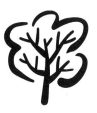

Trevira
See *polyester*.

Trichloroethane
Commonly used as a *solvent* and cleaning agent in spot removers, fabric cleaners, *paints* and *varnish* removers, degreasers, typewriter correction fluids and *insecticides*. Also used as an *aerosol propellant*. Restrictions on levels in drinking *water*.

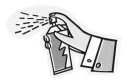

Trichloroethylene
A *solvent* used to remove grease from *textiles* and metal parts, and in the extraction of vegetable oils. Restrictions on levels in drinking *water*.

Triethanolamine
Also known as triolamine, trolamine and TEA. Used in personal care products (e.g. skin lotions, eye gels, moisturisers, shampoos, shaving foams etc.). Under certain circumstances may produce *nitrosamines*.

Trihalomethanes
Also known as TTHMs. Chloroform iodoform and bromoform are TTHMs. Used to make other chemicals. Can also be formed in small amounts when *chlorine* is added to water, as an interaction between the chlorine and natural organic matter. May be found in drinking *water*, bottled water and *swimming pool water*. Chloroform no longer used as an *anaesthetic*.

Trimethylsiloxysilicate
Also known as homosalate. Used as a waterproofing agent in *sunscreen preparations*.

Triphenyl Phosphate
A flame retardant added to many *plastics* such as televisions and computer monitors. When the appliance heats up in use, small amounts of this chemical vaporise into the air.

TTHMs
See *trihalomethanes*.

Turmeric
A spice used in curries, etc. Also used in some processed food as a colouring agent. Also see *curcumin*.

Turpentine

Volatile essential oils obtained from trees (mainly pine). Used in *cosmetics*, polishes including *shoe polish*, *varnishes*, thinners for *paints*, pine scented products, indigestion mixtures, and heat-generating skin rubs. Used to make *colophony*.

Tyramine

Foods rich in tyramine include red *wine*, fermented and aged products, over-ripe fruit, meat and fish dishes prepared more than 48 hours before consumption, some cheeses and *yeast extract*. Can trigger cluster *headaches* in some people, but usually not an allergic reaction, but because susceptible people have lower levels of a platelet enzyme (phenolsulphotransferase) that breaks tyramine down.

U

Unperfumed

This means that the product has no noticeable smell, but *perfumes* may have been added to mask the smell of other ingredients. See also *perfume*.

Unscented

See *unperfumed*.

Urine

Urine from mice, rats, guinea-pigs and hamsters can be a problem. In pet animals the bedding becomes contaminated, and then the activity of the animal releases large amounts of urine proteins into the air. Cans, bottles and packing may be contaminated with rat urine from storage in supermarket warehouses.

V

Vaccines

As well as the active ingredient, there is likely to be a preservative such as *thimerosal, phenol, formaldehyde, aluminium hydroxide, 2-phenoxyethanol* or benzethonium chloride.

Vanilla

A natural *flavouring* coming from the vanilla pod. In same botanical family as orchids. Widely used in confectionary and desserts, including foods that are not obviously vanilla flavoured such as *chocolate* products and some breakfast cereals. Also used as a perfume in personal care products and cosmetics. See also *vanillin*.

Vanillin

A synthetic replica of *vanilla* used as a *flavouring* in *chocolate*, cakes, desserts, and yoghurt. Also used in some *perfumes*.

Varnish

Contains a variety of chemicals (such as *abietic acid* and *methanol*); used to give a hard glossy surface.

Vegetable Fat

See *vegetable oil. hydrogenated vegetable oil* and *margarine*.

Vegetable Oil

Can be made from various oils and can vary from time to time depending on which ones happen to be cheapest for the manufacturer at that time. Oils extracted from numerous sources - *corn, soya* beans, *peanuts*, cottonseeds, safflower seeds, *rape/canola* and *sunflower* seeds. Seeds are collected when ripe and then

cleaned. Unless the oil is cold-pressed, the seeds are cooked (to free the oil for efficient pressing) and then dried.
The mixture is then pressed using a continuous screw press, filtered, and allowed to settle. More oil is extracted from the sediment using *solvents* such as *hexane* or *heptane*. The solvent is then removed by distillation. Sold as 'vegetable oil' or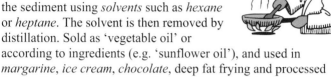
according to ingredients (e.g. 'sunflower oil'), and used in *margarine*, *ice cream*, *chocolate*, deep fat frying and processed foods. See also *hydrogenated vegetable oil*, *acrylamide* and *margarine*.

Vehicle Exhaust Fumes
Exhaust gases include nitrous oxide, *nitrogen dioxide, formaldehyde, benzene, sulphur dioxide, hydrogen sulphide*, carbon dioxide, *carbon monoxide, ethylene dichloride* and *methanol*. Petrol engines produce more *carbon monoxide* but much less soot (carbon) 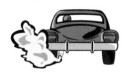 than diesel engines. Some cases of car/automobile sickness are caused by sensitivity to either petrol or diesel fumes. Once this has been corrected the problem disappears. See also *particulate matter*.

Vermouth
Wine flavoured with herbs, spices, barks and flowers. Each manufacturer has own secret recipe.

Vinegar
Made from different substances depending on the type of vinegar, plus *yeast* and Acetobacter aceti bacteria. Can be made directly from *sugar*, or by first converting the sugar into *alcohol* and then turning the alcohol into vinegar. Malt vinegar, made by fermentation of *barley malt* or other cereals. Cider vinegar from *apples*. Balsamic vinegar from white sweet *grapes* aged over several years in wood

barrels (oak, cherry, chestnut, mulberry, acacia, juniper or ash). See also *acetic acid*.

Vinyl Acetate
Found in water-based latex *paints* and in *adhesives* for *paper* and wood.

Vinylbenzene
See styrene.

Vinyl Chloride
Used to make *polyvinyl chloride*. Can be formed when other substances such as *trichloroethane, trichloroethylene*, and *tetrachloroethylene* are broken down. Used in furniture, wall coverings, car/automobile upholstery, and car/automotive parts.

Vinylidene Chloride
Produced in the manufacture of *trichloroethane, perchloroethylene*, and *trichloroethylene*. Low levels detected in the air, particularly in industrialised areas.

Viscose
See *rayon*.

Vitamin B2
See *riboflavin*.

Vitamin C
See *ascorbic acid*.

Vitamin E
Also known as E306. A natural *antioxidant* extracted from *soya* bean oil, wheat germ or cottonseed. Found in meat pies, sausages, mayonnaise, *margarine*, and dessert toppings. Also found in *nutritional supplements*.

VOCs

See *volatile organic compounds*.

Vodka

A clear alcoholic spirit originating in Russia that is made from *grain*.

Volatile Organic Compounds

Also known as VOC's. Lightweight organic molecules that easily evaporate into the air. VOC's include *formaldehyde*, *benzene*, *toluene*, *xylene*, *styrene*, etc. Levels of VOC's in new homes are twice as high as those built a decade ago. Currently no standard for the safe limit for VOC's in the UK, but one study found that one in twenty homes that are less than a year old has at least twice the Australian safe limit for VOC's. ('New Scientist' March 8th 2001). Found in many household cleaning agents, personal care products, *pesticides*, *paints*, hobby products, *dry cleaning*, *aerosol* sprays, *adhesives*, and *solvents*.

W

Wasabi

Made from the root of a plant related to horseradish. Used in Japanese cuisine, particularly sushi.

Washing Up Liquid

Similar ingredients to *detergents* and *dishwasher powders*. Traces of washing up liquid will often remain on *cutlery* and *crockery* and cause problems for sensitive individuals.

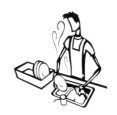

Washing Powder

See *detergent*.

Wasp Sting

A potentially severe allergy that can cause *anaphylactic shock*. Some people believe that wasp sting is alkaline and *bee sting* is acid, but scientific understanding does not support this. Information on the Keele University Arboretum web site, for example, says 'Contrary to popular belief a wasp sting is neutral NOT alkaline with a pH of 6.8 to 6.9 therefore the application of an acid will do no good.' Nevertheless you will see this belief frequently in books and on the web. This has implications for allergy work because it is sometimes said that correcting a wasp sting allergy will correct a reaction to all alkaline stings.

Water

Common pollutants include fertilisers, weed killers, industrial chemicals, metals, hormones (e.g. oestrogens) and bacteria. Also *chlorine*, fluoride and *aluminium sulphate* added as part of processing drinking water. *Trihalomethanes*, *bromodichloromethane* and *dibromoacetic acid* may be found as a result of the chlorination process. Modern plumbing is usually made from *polybutylene*, *copper* and *polyvinyl chloride*, but in some areas still some lead pipes.

Water Colour Paints

Consist of ground pigments and *gum Arabic*.

Water Filters

The simplest water purifying filters are made from carbon (mainly from coal, *coconut* or bone), sometimes with the addition of *silver*. Reverse osmosis water filters usually have a *plastic* membrane and a carbon block.

Water Purifiers
See *water filters*.

Water Softeners
Domestic water softening systems are based on a *plastic resin* (cross linked *polystyrene*) charged with sodium.

Waxes
Soft water-repellant substances. Used in polishes, electrical insulation, *fabrics*, *leather*, *drugs* and coatings on *paper*.

Weed Pollens
Weeds can be very allergenic, as their *pollen* is often small and insignificant, relying on dispersal in the air. Plantain, mugwort and *ragweed* are common problems in areas where they grow. In the UK most weed pollens occur between the end of June and the beginning of September, but can start as early as February. See appendix 3 for a pollens calendar.

Wheat
Many people who are sensitive to wheat assume that the problem lies in the *gluten*, but may be other constituents in the wheat. Wheat is found in *bread* (including some *rye* bread), biscuits/cookies and other *baked goods*, in *pasta* and breakfast cereals, many sausages and cold meats, hamburgers, and as a thickener in processed foods.

Whey
Whey is a protein derived from *milk*. The other main milk protein is *casein*. Ricotta and Gjetost cheeses are made from whey. Whey is altered by high heat, and so people sensitive to whey may be able to tolerate evaporated, boiled, or UHT milk and milk powder.

Whiskey
See *whisky*.

Whisky
The grains used vary depending on the country of origin, but may contain *corn*, *rye*, *wheat* and *barley*, as well as *yeast*. May be matured in oak barrels or old sherry barrels.

White Paraffin
Also known as petrolatum album and white petrolatum. Used in ointments. See also *paraffin*.

White Wine
See *wine*.

Wine
Made from *grapes*, *yeast* and various additives, (e.g. potassium tartrate, *citric acid, tartaric acid, sorbic acid, diammonium phosphate, sulphur dioxide, gelatine, egg albumen* etc.) May be matured in wood barrels. Some people are only allergic to one type of wine (red or white). Red wine is not made from red grapes and white wine from white grapes as is popularly supposed. Red wines are made by fermenting the pips, skins and sometimes the stems (as well as the fruit). *Tannin* used in red wine to preserve it. High levels of *tyramine* in red wine. Where a person is only sensitive to white wines it is possible that they are reacting to *bentonite*, used extensively for refining white wine, but rarely for red. White and sweet wines also contain more *sulphur dioxide* than red ones. Both red and white wine may contain *histamine*; the younger the wine the higher the histamine content is likely to be.

Wood Alcohol
See *methanol*.

Wood Distillate
A flavouring used in smoked foods.

Wool

A very common allergen. See also *lanolin*.

Wool Alcohol

See *lanolin*.

Worcestershire Sauce

A bottled condiment made from anchovies, onions and *garlic*.

X

Xanthan Gum

Also known as E415. A *stabiliser* commonly used in *soft drinks*, mustard, salad dressings, mayonnaise, dips, sauces, confectionery, hot chocolate drinks and cereal bars. Also used in personal care products such as moisturisers, cleansing lotions, foundation and *toothpastes*.

Xylene

A chemical used in cleaners, *paints*, *lacquers*, *adhesives* in flooring material, *nail polish*, *varnish* removers, *cement* and damp start products sprayed on car/automobile engines. Also used in *insecticides*.

Xylitol

Also known as E967. A sweetener produced from birch trees with a slightly minty flavour. Used in *chewing gum* and mouth freshener mints.

Y

Yeast

Yeasts can be divided into *baker's yeast*, *brewer's yeast*, or nutritional yeasts (e.g. torula). A person can have problems with one type but not the others. Very common allergens.

Yeast Concentrate

See *yeast extract*.

Yeast Extract

Yeast extract is derived from *brewer's yeast*.

Yellow Jacket

See *wasp sting*.

Yoghurt

Traditional yoghurt culture contains a mix of Lactobacillus bulgaricus and Streptococcus thermophilus bacteria. Bio-yoghurts also contain Lactobacillus acidophilus and Bifidobacterium bifidum. Yoghurt that is sold as pasteurised, sterilised or UHT may not contain any live bacteria. Usually well tolerated by people who are *lactose* intolerant.

Z

Zest
From the skin of citrus fruit. Used in *baked goods*.
Zinc
A metal found in *dental amalgam*, some solders, some *coins*, *brass*, used as a dye in *tattooing*. Exposure also occurs where galvanised iron is deteriorating and as a result of industrial *pollution*.

Zylon
See *polypropylene*.

Appendix 1: Classification Of Food Additives

E Number	Name	FD & C	C.I. Number	Other
E100	curcumin		C.I. 75300	
E101	riboflavin			
E102	tartrazine	FD & C Yellow 5	C.I. 19140	food yellow 4
E104	quinoline yellow		C.I. 47005	food yellow 13
E110	sunset yellow	FD & C Yellow 6	C.I. 15985	food yellow 3
E120	carminic acid		C.I. 75470	natural red 4
E122	carmoisine		C.I. 14720	food red 3
E123	amaranth	FD & C Red 2	C.I. 16185	food red 9
E124	ponceau 4R		C.I. 16255	food red 7
E127	erythrosine	FD & C Red 3	C.I. 45430	food red 14
E128	red 2G		C.I. 18050	
E129	allura red AC	FD & C Red 40	C.I. 16035	food red 17
E131	patent blue V		C.I. 42051	food blue 5
E132	indigo carmine	FD & C Blue 2	C.I. 73015	food blue 1
E133	brilliant blue FCF	FD & C Blue 1	C.I. 42090	food blue 2
does not have	fast green FCF	FD & C Green 3	C.I. 42053	food green 3
E140	chlorophyll		C.I. 75810	
E141	copper complexes		C.I. 75810	
E142	green S		C.I. 44090	food green S
E150a to d	caramel			

E Number	Name	FD & C	C.I. Number	Other
E151	black PN		C.I. 28440	
E160	carotenoids			
E160a	beta carotene		C.I. 75130	
E160b	annatto		C.I. 75120	
E160c	capsanthin			
E161	carotenoids			
E161b	lutein		C.I. 75135	
E162	betanin			
E163	anthocyanins			
E171	titanium dioxide		C.I. 77891	
E173	aluminium		C.I. 77000	
E174	Silver		C.I. 77820	
E200	sorbic acid			
E202	potassium sorbate			
E210	benzoic acid			
E211	sodium benzoate			
E212	potassium			
E220	sulphur dioxide			
E222	sodium hydrogen			
E223	sodium			
E231	orthophenyl			
E250	sodium nitrite			
E251	sodium nitrate			

E Number	Name	FD & C	C.I. Number	Other
E260	acetic acid			
E270	lactic acid			
E300	ascorbic acid			
E306	vitamin E			
E311	octyl gallate			
E320	butylated			
E321	butylated			
E322	lecithin			
E330	citric acid			
E334	tartaric acid			
E338	phosphoric acid			
E341	calcium			
E343	magnesium			
E400	alginic acid			
E401	sodium alginate			
E404	calcium alginate			
E407	carageenan			
E410	locust bean gum			
E412	guar gum			
E413	gum tragacanth			
E414	gum Arabic			
E415	xanthan gum			
E420	sorbitol			

E Number	Name	FD & C	C.I. Number	Other
E421	mannitol			
E422	glycerol			
E432	polysorbate 20			
E433	polysorbate 80			
E440(a)	pectin			
E450(b)	sodium			
E450(i)	disodium			
E466	sodium			
E471	mono- and di-			
E475	polyglycerol esters			
E476	polyglycerol			
E491	sorbitan			
E500	sodium			
E509	calcium chloride			
E541	sodium aluminium			
E621	monosodium			
E920	L-cysteine			
E950	acesulfame-K			
E951	aspartame			
E967	xylitol			

Appendix 2: Food Families

This is not a totally comprehensive list but covers most of the commonly eaten foods:

Banana
Banana, plantain

Birch
Filbert, hazelnut

Buckwheat
Buckwheat, garden sorrel, rhubarb

Cashew
Cashew nut, mango, pistachio (also poison ivy)

Citrus
Orange, lemon, grapefruit, tangerine, clementine, ugly fruit, satsuma, lime, angostura, kumquat, mandarin

Composite
Lettuce, chicory, sesame, sunflower, safflower, burdock, dandelion, camomile, artichoke (globe and Jerusalem), pyrethrum, absinthe, salsify, vermouth, ragweed, yarrow, endive

Euphorbia
Cassava, tapioca

Fungi Or Moulds
Baker's yeast, brewer's yeast, mushroom, truffle, chanterelle, blue cheese, vinegar, antibiotics

Gooseberry
Red currant, black currant, gooseberry

Goosefoot
Spinach, chard, sugar beet, lamb's lettuce / quarters, thistle, beetroot

Gourd
Melon, cucumber, squash, gherkin, courgette, marrow, pumpkin

Grape
Wine, champagne, brandy, sherry, raisin, currant (dried), sultana, cream of tartar, wine vinegar

Grasses/Grains
Wheat, corn, barley, oats, millet, cane sugar, bamboo shoots, rice, rye (note that buckwheat is *not* a member of the grass family)

Heath
Cranberry, blueberry, huckleberry, wintergreen

Laurel
Avocado, bay, camphor, cinnamon, laurel, sassafras

Legume / Pulses
Acacia, alfalfa, gum Arabic, pea, carob, cassia, chick pea, green bean, guar gum, haricot bean, kidney bean, lentil, liquorice, lima bean, locust bean gum, mung bean, navy bean, peanut, pinto bean, soya bean, textured vegetable protein (TVP), string bean, tamarind, tragacanth gum, urd flour (used in Indian cookery)

Lily
Onion, asparagus, chives, leek, garlic, sarsaparilla, shallot

Mallow
Cottonseed, okra

Mint
Mint, peppermint, basil, marjoram, oregano, sage, rosemary,
savoury, thyme, balm

Morning Glory
Sweet potato, yam

Mulberry
Breadfruit, fig, hops, mulberry

Mustard
Broccoli, cabbage, cauliflower, Brussels sprouts, collard, horseradish, kohlrabi, radish, swede, turnip, watercress, mustard, cress,
watercress, rutabaga, kale

Myrtle
Allspice, cloves, eucalyptus, guava

Nightshade
Potato, tomato, tobacco, aubergine/eggplant, cayenne, bell pepper,
chilli, sweet pepper, paprika, pimento

Nutmeg
Mace, nutmeg, brazil nut

Palm
Coconut, date, sago

Parsley
Carrot, parsley, dill, celery, fennel, parsnip, aniseed, angelica,
celeriac, caraway, coriander, cumin, sweet cicely

Pulses Or Legumes
Pea, chick pea, soy bean (hence TVP), lentils, liquorice, peanut,
kidney bean, string bean, haricot bean, mung bean, alfalfa

Rose
Apple, pear, quince, almond, apricot, cherry, peach, plum, sloe, blackberry, loganberry, raspberry, strawberry, boysenberry, dewberry, nectarine, prune, bilberry, blueberry, huckleberry, cranberry (this family is sometimes sub-divided further)

Sterculia
Chocolate, cocoa, cola nut

Walnut
Walnut, pecan, butternut, hickory

The following foods have no *commonly* eaten relatives:
juniper, pineapple, vanilla, black pepper, chestnut, maple, lychee, kiwi fruit, tea, coffee, papaya, ginseng, olive

There appear to be several different ways of classifying animals. Here is one possibility.

Ruminants
Cattle (beef), milk and dairy products, mutton, lamb, goat, deer (venison)

Duck
Duck, goose

Game Birds
Pheasant, quail, turkey (turkey also gets listed under poultry)

Poultry
Chicken, eggs, turkey (turkey also gets listed under game birds)

Swine
Pork, bacon, lard (dripping), ham, sausage

Codfish
Haddock, cod, ling (saith), coley, hake

Crustaceans
Lobster, prawn, shrimp, crab, crayfish

Flatfish
Dab, flounder, halibut, turbot, sole, plaice

Herring
Pilchard, sardine, herring, rollmop

Mackerel
Tuna, bonito, tuny, mackerel, skipjack

Molluscs
Snail, abalone, squid, clam, mussel, oyster, scallop

Salmon
Salmon, trout, bass, catfish, perch, pike

The following foods have no *commonly* eaten relatives:
anchovy, sturgeon (caviar), rabbit

Appendix 3: Pollen Calendar

The exact dates will vary depending on the weather in that year and the country, but this regional pollen calendar will give some indications of when particular types of pollen are most prevalent.

	Australia	Europe	Mid West USA	North East USA	Western USA
Trees	October to beginning of May	February to July	April to beginning of June	April to July	January to June
Grasses	October to beginning of June	April to beginning of September	June to September	April to September	All year
Weeds	September to April	End of February to beginning of October	July to beginning of October	August to October	April to August

This information is taken from a much more detailed pollen calendar at:
http://www.hon.ch/Library/Theme/Allergy/Glossary/calendar.html

Appendix 4: For Practitioners & Students

GENERAL CONSIDERATIONS

From time to time I meet practitioners involved in allergy testing who are testing only the 'standard' foods, such as milk and wheat. This will help many people, but there are many others whose allergies need a broader approach. Helping some people needs painstaking detective work, but the results are well worth the effort.

Do remember when you look at the A to Z section of this book, that I have tried to make it as comprehensive as I can, and that some of the information will only be relevant occasionally.

Whatever system of testing you are using, it is important to be clear what you mean by 'allergy', 'intolerance' and 'sensitivity'. In particular when you talk to people who are medically trained, you need to be explicit if you are using a different definition than the accepted medical ones for the terms 'allergy' and 'tolerance'.

It seems likely that there are several mechanisms involved in what the general public refer to as 'allergies'. If this is the case, there is unlikely to be one simple test that will detect all instances. In kinesiology terms, for instance, this means that there needs to be more than one protocol for detecting problems, and more than one treatment.

This may explain why the whole area of 'allergy testing' is so fraught with difficulty. In the 1980's I used kinesiology to test hundreds of people for allergies. Some of these people had also been tested using conventional medical procedures. Often I found that I came up with completely different results. It could indicate that one of us (or even both!) was wrong, or it could be that different types of reaction were being tested. If I came up with the same culprits as had been established by medical testing, I used to tell the client (jokingly) that I must have made a mistake. Many magazines have run features where a journalist has been sent to a variety of people for allergy testing, and there is no consistency in the results. It is likely that some of this is as a result of bad testing, but it may also indicate that practitioners (medical and complementary) are not necessarily testing the same thing.

OBTAINING TEST SAMPLES

When I was working as a practitioner and extensively involved in allergy testing, I asked clients to bring things in for testing. I also had samples of actual substances in jars, bottles and plastic bags. I found test kits extremely useful, and I developed many of these myself.

Getting Clients To Bring Things

It is a good idea to ask a new client to bring things with them to their initial appointment. Do not leave it up to them what to bring but give them a list. What you ask them to bring depends on what you have available in your office. If you do not have test kits, you might want to ask clients to bring perishable foods such as meat, fruit and vegetables and dairy items. My own experience of doing this was that many people would turn up for their appointment with only a few of the things I had asked them to bring, so with time I came to reply more on test kits. Even if you use test kits it is a good idea to ask people to bring any *drugs* and *nutritional supplements* that they are currently taking, samples of *pet hair*, etc. I usually ask people to bring in their drinking water as it can vary so much. Even when houses are next to each other the water may be different because the plumbing may be different. Also if people work away from home, ask them to bring in the water they drink at work.

Less obvious samples include 'dust' from extractor fans and the contents of the vacuum cleaner. Both of these samples will give a mixture of substances that are encountered by people living/working in that area.

If a person's symptoms are worse in a particular room or area, and you cannot identify the exact problem, you can still correct the problem (using kinesiology etc.) by taking a 'sample' of the area. To do this ask the client to put a small glass bowl containing water in the area and leave for 24 hours. They then bring the water in for testing – they can transfer the water from the bowl to a clean jar for ease of carriage. The water will contain *pollution*, *dust*, hair, fibres, *pollens*, and, possibly, energy vibrations – a unique picture of a specific place.

Physical Substances
You can collect things to keep ready for testing in your office. Be sure to label everything clearly. I added to my collection by keeping some of the substances that clients brought in (e.g. pet hair, washing powder, etc.)

Test Kits
There is a wide range of homeopathic/radionic test kits available from different companies. Life-Work Potential has over 60 different kits, including many suitable for allergy testing. The advantage of these kits is that you can easily test a wide range of substances. Also, when using test kits, it is possible to test blind (without the client knowing what you are testing) or even double-blind (where neither you nor the client know).

In my experience using kinesiology for allergy testing, I have found problems if I test substances that are in plastic containers or wrappings. For a more detailed discussion of this and other information on allergy testing see my book 'Energy Mismatch'.

My book 'Verbal Testing Skills For Kinesiologists' also has a section on allergy and intolerance testing.

References

Linda Gamblin   The Allergy Bible

Reader's Digest   The Stomach and Digestive System

Peter Parish   Medicines A Guide For Everyone

D.W.A. Sharp   The Penguin Dictionary of Chemistry

P. Cox & P. Brusseau   Secret Ingredients

Niels Mygind et al   Essential Allergy

Women's Environmental Network *Getting Lippy*

Ken Digby of NT Labs Ltd.
for information on water purification.

Carla Payne and Douglas Clarke of Seven Wives
for information on soap and personal care products.

York Laboratory, UK
for information on ELISA testing
www.yorktest.com

Sean Tume, Moana, Australia
for information on the EAV system of testing
http://www.energymedcollege.com

Mark Varey 'Allergy testing In the Laboratory' Positive Health
http://www.positivehealth.com/permit/Articles/Allergy/varey15.htm
for information on cytotoxic and RAST testing

http://www.yorks.karoo.net/aerosol/link4.htm
information on aerosol propellants

http://www.ibas.btinternet.co.uk/
for information on asbestos

http://www.ncia-ltd.org.uk/Page1.asp
for information on cavity wall insulation

http://www.tclayton.demon.co.uk/metal.html
for information on metals in coins worldwide

http://www.royalmint.com/talk/default.asp
for information on metals in British Coins

http://www.fhi.org/en/RH/Pubs/booksReports/latexcondom/recentad
vances.htm
for information on condoms

http://www.ineedcoffee.com/99/06/decaf/
for information on decaffeination

http://www.soapdetergents.com/doc/doc_ing.asp?IDDOC=2
for information on detergents

http://www.cleaning101.com/dishwash/dishwashing_fact_sheet4.ht
ml
for information on dishwasher powders

http://www.fda.gov/ora/inspect_ref/iom/APPENDICES/appA2.html
for information on food additives

http://www.fao.org/documents/show_cdr.asp?url_file=/docrep/V503 0E/V5030E0q.htm
FAO site dealing with fruit and vegetable processing

http://householdproducts.nlm.nih.gov/
US National Institutes of Health database of household products

http://meyergs.com/id60.htm
for information on hazardous substances in household products

http://www.madsci.org/posts/archives/dec97/879637779.Ot.r.html
for information on leather tanning

http://pubs.acs.org/cen/whatstuff/stuff/7728scit2.html
for ingredients in lipsticks

http://www.fibersource.com/
for information on man-made fabrics

http://www.cip.ukcentre.com/marg1.htm
for information on margarine manufacture

http://www.margarine.org/
for information on margarine manufacture

http://www.americanrecycler.com/09west02.html
for information on mattresses

http://www.dehs.umn.edu/iaq/fungus/glossary.html
for information of indoor and outdoor moulds

http://www.foe.co.uk/pubsinfo/briefings/html/19971215150024.html
for information on paper

http://www.greatvistachemicals.com/
for information on various chemicals, particularly those related to personal care products and cosmetics.

http://www.ulta.com/control/qa_ingredients
for information on ingredients in personal care products and cosmetics

http://www.dermaxime.com/index.htm
for information on ingredients in personal care products and cosmetics

http://www.dermaxime.com/index.htm
for information on ingredients in personal care products and cosmetics

http://www.plastics.org.nz/page.asp?id=585
for information on plastics

http://www.psrc.usm.edu/macrog/pe.htm
for information on polyethylene, PVC, etc.

http://www.iisrp.com/synthetic-rubber.html
for information on rubber

http://www.adenna.com/rc_Glossary.htm
for information on rubber gloves

http://www.dermadoctor.com/pages/newsletter113.asp?WID=%7B3 2B0374A-57B6-42BC-8428-E28DA693DC81%7D
for information on tattoo dyes

http://www.saveyoursmile.com/toothpaste/toothpaste-c.html
for information on toothpaste ingredients

http://www.epa.gov/
The web site of the US Environmental Protection Agency

http://www.atsdr.cdc.gov/
The web site of the Agency For Toxic Substance & Disease Registry